Mimics, Pearls, and Pitfalls of Head and Neck Imaging

Editors

GUL MOONIS

DANIEL T. GINAT

NEUROIMAGING CLINICS OF NORTH AMERICA

www.neuroimaging.theclinics.com

Consulting Editor
SURESH K. MUKHERJI

May 2022 • Volume 32 • Number 2

ELSEVIER

1600 John F. Kennedy Boulevard • Suite 1800 • Philadelphia, Pennsylvania, 19103-2899

http://www.neuroimaging.theclinics.com

NEUROIMAGING CLINICS OF NORTH AMERICA Volume 32, Number 2
February 2022 ISSN 1052-5149, ISBN 13: 978-0-323-84854-1

Editor: John Vassallo (j.vassallo@elsevier.com)
Developmental Editor: Karen Solomon

Neuroimaging Clinics of North America (ISSN 1052-5149) is published quarterly by Elsevier Inc., 360 Park Avenue South, New York, NY 10010-1710. Months of issue are February, May, August, and November. Business and editorial offices: 1600 John F. Kennedy Blvd., Suite 1800, Philadelphia, PA 19103-2899. Business and editorial offices: 6277 Sea Harbor Drive, Orlando, FL 32887-4800. Periodicals postage paid at New York, NY, and additional mailing offices. Subscription prices are USD 401 per year for US individuals, USD 932 per year for US institutions, USD 100 per year for US students and residents, USD 469 per year for Canadian individuals, USD 946 per year for Canadian institutions, USD 546 per year for international individuals, USD 946 per year for international institutions, USD 100 per year for Canadian students and residents and USD 260 per year for foreign students and residents. To receive student/resident rate, orders must be accompanied by name of affiliated institution, date of term, and the *signature* of program/residency coordinator on institution letterhead. Orders will be billed at individual rate until proof of status is received. Foreign air speed delivery is included in all *Clinics* subscription prices. All prices are subject to change without notice. POSTMASTER: Send address changes to *Neuroimaging Clinics of North America*, Elsevier Health Sciences Division, Subscription **Customer Service, 3251 Riverport Lane, Maryland Heights, MO 63043. Telephone: 1-800-654-2452 (U.S. and Canada); 314-447-8871 (outside U.S. and Canada). Fax: 314-447-8029. E-mail: journalscustomerservice-usa@elsevier.com (for print support); journalsonlinesupport-usa@elsevier.com (for online support).**

Reprints. For copies of 100 or more of articles in this publication, please contact the Commercial Reprints Department, Elsevier Inc., 360 Park Avenue South, New York, NY 10010-1710. Tel.: 212-633-3874; Fax: 212-633-3820; E-mail: reprints@elsevier.com.

Neuroimaging Clinics of North America is covered by *Excerpta Medical/EMBASE,* the RSNA Index of Imaging Literature, *MEDLINE/PubMed (Index Medicus),* MEDLINE/MEDLARS, SciSearch, Research Alert, and Neuroscience Citation Index.

PROGRAM OBJECTIVE

The goal of *Neuroimaging Clinics of North America* is to keep practicing radiologists and radiology residents up to date with current clinical practice in radiology by providing timely articles reviewing the state of the art in patient care.

TARGET AUDIENCE

Practicing radiologists, radiology residents, and other healthcare professionals who utilize neuroimaging findings to provide patient care.

LEARNING OBJECTIVES

Upon completion of this activity, participants will be able to:

1. Review the normal anatomy and physiology and anatomic variants of the head and neck to help establish a systematic approach to recognizing mimickers and pitfalls when using imaging as a diagnostic and interpretation tool for head and neck disorders before and after treatment.
2. Discuss artifacts and technical difficulties, such as taking a multidisciplinary approach to avoid interfering with imaging interpretation, unneeded imaging, and assisting in the proper therapy of head and neck disorders.
3. Recognize mimickers, artifacts, and their causes, which are related to the patient, hardware, and signal processing and can lead to errors in diagnosing and treating head and neck disorders.

ACCREDITATION

The Elsevier Office of Continuing Medical Education (EOCME) is accredited by the Accreditation Council for Continuing Medical Education (ACCME) to provide continuing medical education for physicians.

The EOCME designates this journal-based CME activity for a maximum of 12 *AMA PRA Category 1 Credit*(s)™. Physicians should claim only the credit commensurate with the extent of their participation in the activity.

All other healthcare professionals requesting continuing education credit for this enduring material will be issued a certificate of participation.

DISCLOSURE OF CONFLICTS OF INTEREST

The EOCME assesses conflict of interest with its instructors, faculty, planners, and other individuals who are in a position to control the content of CME activities. All relevant conflicts of interest that are identified are thoroughly vetted by EOCME for fair balance, scientific objectivity, and patient care recommendations. EOCME is committed to providing its learners with CME activities that promote improvements or quality in healthcare and not a specific proprietary business or a commercial interest.

The planning committee, staff, authors, and editors listed below have identified no financial relationships or relationships to products or devices they or their spouse/life partner have with commercial interest related to the content of this CME activity:

Ahmad Amer, BS; Ariel Botwin, MD; Paul M. Bunch, MD; Felice D'Arco, MD; Edward J. Escott, MD; Daniel T. Ginat, MD, MS; Mari Hagiwara, MD; Jeffrey H. Huang, MD; Jason Michael Johnson, MD; Amy Juliano, MD; June Kim, MD; Pradeep Kuttysankaran; Gul Moonis, MD; Suresh K. Mukherji, MD, MBA, FACR; Charles Pierce, MD, MS; Steffen Sammet, MD, PhD; Doreen Thomas-Payne, MSN, BSN, RN, PMHNP-BC; Lorenzo Ugga, MD, PhD; John Vassallo; Randy Yeh, MD

The planning committee, staff, authors, and editors listed below have identified financial relationships or relationships to products or devices they or their spouse/life partner have with commercial interest related to the content of this CME activity:

Hillary R. Kelly, MD: Researcher: Bayer AG

Emily L. Marshall, PhD: Consultant: Bayer AG

UNAPPROVED/OFF-LABEL USE DISCLOSURE

The EOCME requires CME faculty to disclose to the participants:

1. When products or procedures being discussed are off-label, unlabelled, experimental, and/or investigational (not US Food and Drug Administration [FDA] approved); and
2. Any limitations on the information presented, such as data that are preliminary or that represent ongoing research, interim analyses, and/or unsupported opinions. Faculty may discuss information about pharmaceutical agents that is outside of FDA-approved labelling. This information is intended solely for CME and is not intended to promote off-label use of these medications. If you have any questions, contact the medical affairs department of the manufacturer for the most recent prescribing information.

TO ENROLL

To enroll in the *Neuroimaging Clinics of North America* Continuing Medical Education program, call customer service at 1-800-654-2452 or sign up online at http://www.theclinics.com/home/cme. The CME program is available to subscribers for an additional annual fee of USD 265.00.

METHOD OF PARTICIPATION

In order to claim credit, participants must complete the following:

1. Complete enrolment as indicated above.
2. Read the activity.
3. Complete the CME Test and Evaluation. Participants must achieve a score of 70% on the test. All CME Tests and Evaluations must be completed online.

CME INQUIRIES/SPECIAL NEEDS

For all CME inquiries or special needs, please contact elsevierCME@elsevier.com.

NEUROIMAGING CLINICS OF NORTH AMERICA

FORTHCOMING ISSUES

August 2022
Neuroimaging Anatomy, Part 1: Brain and Skull
Tarik F. Massoud, *Editor*

November 2022
Neuroimaging Anatomy, Part 2: Head, Neck, and Spine
Tarik F. Massoud, *Editor*

February 2023
Central Nervous System Infections
Tchoyoson Lim Choie Cheio, *Editor*

RECENT ISSUES

February 2022
Imaging of the Post Treatment Head and Neck
Prashant Raghavan, Robert E. Morales, and Sugoto Mukherjee, *Editors*

November 2021
Skull Base Neuroimaging
Steve E.J. Connor, *Editor*

August 2021
Thyroid and Parathyroid Imaging
Salmaan Ahmed and James Matthew Debnam, *Editors*

SERIES OF RELATED INTEREST

Advances in Clinical Radiology
Available at: Advancesinclinicalradiology.com
MRI Clinics of North America
Available at: MRI.theclinics.com
PET Clinics
Available at: https://www.pet.theclinics.com/
Radiologic Clinics of North America
Available at: Radiologic.theclinics.com

THE CLINICS ARE AVAILABLE ONLINE!
Access your subscription at:
www.theclinics.com

NEUROIMAGING CLINICS OF NORTH AMERICA

Contributors

CONSULTING EDITOR

SURESH K. MUKHERJI, MD, MBA, FACR
Clinical Professor of Radiology and Radiation Oncology, University of Illinois, Peoria, Illinois, USA; Robert Wood Johnson Medical School, Rutgers University, New Brunswick, New Jersey, USA; Faculty, Otolaryngology Head Neck Surgery, Michigan State University, Farmington Hills, Michigan, USA; National Director of Head and Neck Radiology, ProScan Imaging, Carmel, Indiana, USA

EDITORS

GUL MOONIS, MD
Professor, Department of Radiology, NYU Langone Medical Center, New York, New York, USA

DANIEL T. GINAT, MD, MS
Director of Head and Neck Imaging, Associate Professor, Department of Radiology, University of Chicago, Chicago, Illinois, USA

AUTHORS

AHMAD AMER, BS
Department of Neuroradiology, The University of Texas MD Anderson Cancer Center, MSIII, Chicago Medical School at Rosalind Franklin University of Medicine and Science, Houston, Texas, USA

ARIEL BOTWIN, MD
Massachusetts General Hospital, Boston, Massachusetts, USA

PAUL M. BUNCH, MD
Assistant Professor, Department of Radiology, Wake Forest School of Medicine, Winston Salem, North Carolina, USA

FELICE D'ARCO, MD
Department of Radiology, Neuroradiology Unit, Great Ormond Street Hospital, London, United Kingdom

EDWARD J. ESCOTT, MD
Department of Radiology, University of Kentucky, Lexington, Kentucky, USA

DANIEL T. GINAT, MD, MS
Director of Head and Neck Imaging, Associate Professor, Department of Radiology, University of Chicago, Chicago, Illinois, USA

MARI HAGIWARA, MD
Department of Radiology, NYU Langone Health, New York, New York, USA

JEFFREY H. HUANG, MD
Department of Radiology, NYU Langone Health, New York, New York, USA

JASON MICHAEL JOHNSON, MD
Department of Neuroradiology, The University of Texas MD Anderson Cancer Center, Houston, Texas, USA

AMY JULIANO, MD
Massachusetts Eye and Ear, Boston, Massachusetts, USA

HILLARY R. KELLY, MD
Assistant Professor, Departments of Radiology, Massachusetts General Hospital, Massachusetts Eye and Ear, Harvard Medical School, Boston, Massachusetts, USA

JUNE KIM, MD
Department of Radiology, University of Kentucky, Lexington, Kentucky, USA

EMILY L. MARSHALL, PhD
Department of Radiology, University of Chicago, Chicago, Illinois, USA

GUL MOONIS, MD
Professor, Department of Radiology, NYU
Langone Medical Center, New York, New York,
USA

CHARLES PIERCE, MD, MS
University of Illinois at Chicago, Chicago,
Illinois, USA

STEFFEN SAMMET, MD, PHD
Department of Radiology, University of
Chicago, Chicago, Illinois, USA

LORENZO UGGA, MD, PhD
Department of Advanced Biomedical
Sciences, University of Naples "Federico II,"
Naples, Italy

RANDY YEH, MD
Department of Radiology, Molecular Imaging
and Therapy Service, Memorial Sloan
Kettering Cancer Center, New York, New
York, USA

Contents

Computed tomography (CT) artifacts are aberrations that usually degrade the image quality of CT images, but occasionally provide insights regarding actual imaging findings. The presence of artifacts can be attributed to various sources, including patient, scanner, and postprocessing factors. Artifacts can lead to diagnostic errors by obscuring findings or by being misinterpreted as actual lesions. This article reviews various types of CT artifacts that can be encountered in the head and neck region and explain how these artifacts may be mitigated. While we cannot fully eliminate the occurrence of CT artifacts, building an awareness of their cause provides reading physicians the tools to detect and read through their presence. Further, this knowledge may be applied to contribute to protocol adjustments to improve a site's overall imaging practice.

A variety of artifacts can be encountered on head and neck MR imaging. These can be patient-related, hardware-related, or signal-processing–related and affect diagnostic quality or mimic pathology. It is necessary to take MR imaging artifacts into consideration when interpreting images. A basic knowledge of MR imaging physics and the potential origin of MR imaging artifacts can help to find solutions to eliminate or reduce the influence of artifacts on image quality by adjusting acquisition parameters appropriately for a better diagnosis.

[18]FDG-PET plays an important role in cancer imaging. However, there are certain challenges with interpreting head and neck [18]FDG-PET. In this article, examples of technical issues that can undermine the interpretation of the scans, normal physiologic activity that can mimic lesions or obscure lesions, and causes of false positives and false negatives on posttreatment cancer imaging are discussed. In addition, suggestions for addressing potential pitfalls on head and neck [18]FDG-PET are highlighted.

Contents

Foreword

Mimics, Pearls, and Pitfalls of Head and Neck Imaging

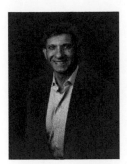

Suresh K. Mukherji, MD, MBA, FACR
Consulting Editor

Years ago, I learned a couple of "tricks" that helped me interpret cross-section imaging of the head and neck. First, ..."draw a line down the middle"... (which was easy when we had "films" and grease pencils!) and compare one side to the other. The head and neck is not completely symmetrical, but looking for large asymmetries helps us identify suspicious areas. The next step was to determine whether that suspicious area was abnormal or whether it represents a normal variation. I still use this approach today and have always appreciated the need to understand normal variation to avoid both "undercalling" and "overcalling" abnormalities. This task becomes even more challenging if you do not routinely interpret head and neck imaging.

It was with this in mind that I invited Drs Gul Moonis and Daniel Ginat to create an issue on Mimics, Pearls, and Pitfalls of Head and Neck Imaging. They have masterfully assembled an wonderful group of head and neck imaging experts who have written state-of-the-art articles on topics that contribute to errors in head and neck radiology and ways to avoid them. The articles cover techniques (CT, MRI, and PET), different anatomical subsites, and normal vascular

variants of the neck. There is also an article specifically devoted to pediatric head and neck. As Drs Moonis and Ginat state in their preface, that while to err is human, the intent of this issue is to help the reader understand and avoid some of the potential mimics and causes of misinterpretation in head and neck radiology.

I would like thank all of the authors for their wonderful contributions to this unique issue. Finally, I would also like to thank Drs Moonis and Ginat. I have known them since they were fellows and have watched their careers evolve into two of the most prolific academic neuroradiologists of their generation. I used to consider them "rising stars," but I can no longer characterize them as such...because they are just "stars"!

Suresh K. Mukherji, MD, MBA, FACR
Marian University
Head and Neck Radiology
ProScan Imaging
Carmel, IN, USA

E-mail address:
sureshmukherji@hotmail.com

neuroimaging.theclinics.com

Preface

Mimics, Pearls, and Pitfalls of Head and Neck Imaging

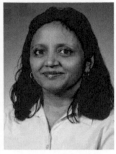
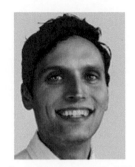

Gul Moonis, MD   Daniel T. Ginat, MD, MS

Editors

Head and neck radiology can be very complex and challenging! Many factors can compromise the successful acquisition and interpretation of head and neck imaging studies. These can be related to the type of imaging modality, anatomical variants, the nature of certain lesions, and factors related to interpreter abilities.

The first step in avoiding pitfalls and mimics is obtaining the most appropriate scan with proper scan parameters and protocols. Efforts should be made to avoid acquiring the scan with artifacts, but it helps to recognize and troubleshoot these if they occur. Once the image is acquired and the radiologist has to review it, one taps into their prior experience and knowledge to parse through the often complex anatomy and pathology. This does not necessarily have to happen in a vacuum. We should consider implementing a systematic approach and consulting all available resources, whether it is the clinical notes, pathology reports, prior imaging, or references in the literature, in order to optimize problem solving. Sometimes these things do not provide additional insights, and even after many years of doing this, we still encounter new challenges. Imaging is often just one part of the puzzle, and further workup can be relied upon.

In this issue of Neuroimaging Clinics, we are privileged to be joined by several head and neck imaging experts who present up-to-date information relevant to radiologists in a systematic manner, addressing various factors that contribute to errors in head and neck radiology and potential mitigation techniques. We have articles based on both techniques (computed tomography, MRI, and PET) and different anatomical subsites of the head and neck, articles on potential postsurgical mimics and implants, an article on normal vascular variants of the neck, and an article on pediatric head and neck pearls and pitfalls. Finally, we have an article on parathyroid imaging pitfalls. While to err is human, we hope that this series of articles will help the reader understand and avoid some of the potential mimics and causes of misinterpretation in head and neck radiology.

We are deeply grateful to Dr Mukherji for the opportunity to create this issue. We hope that this collection of articles will serve as useful references for practicing radiologists in both academic and private practice settings.

Gul Moonis, MD
Department of Radiology
NYU Langone Medical Center
222 E 41st Street
New York, NY 10017, USA

Daniel T. Ginat, MD, MS
Department of Radiology
University of Chicago
5841 S Maryland Avenue
Chicago, IL 60637, USA

E-mail addresses:
Gul.moonis@nyulangone.org (G. Moonis)
ginatd01@gmail.com (D.T. Ginat)

Neuroimag Clin N Am 32 (2022) xv
https://doi.org/10.1016/j.nic.2022.02.005
1052-5149/22/© 2022 Published by Elsevier Inc.

Computed Tomography Imaging Artifacts in the Head and Neck Region
Pitfalls and Solutions

Emily L. Marshall, PhD, Daniel T. Ginat, MD, MS*, Steffen Sammet, MD, PhD

KEYWORDS

- Computed Tomography (CT) • Imaging • Artifacts • Head • Neck

KEY POINTS

- Artifacts in CT can degrade image quality by making diagnoses difficult.
- The underlying causes of individual CT artifacts are identified and discussed.
- Potential solutions are provided toward the elimination of CT artifacts.
- Being familiar with CT artifacts and the underlying physics can help optimize interpretation of head and neck imaging.

INTRODUCTION

Computed tomography (CT) artifacts are aberrations that usually degrade the image quality of CT images, but occasionally provide insights regarding actual imaging findings. The presence of artifacts can be attributed to various sources, including patient, scanner, and postprocessing factors. Artifacts can lead to diagnostic errors by obscuring findings or by being misinterpreted as actual lesions. This article reviews various types of CT artifacts that can be encountered in the head and neck region and explain how these artifacts may be mitigated. While we cannot fully eliminate the occurrence of CT artifacts, building an awareness of their cause provides reading physicians the tools to detect and read through their presence. Further, this knowledge may be applied to contribute to protocol adjustments to improve a site's overall imaging practice.

COMPUTED TOMOGRAPHY ARTIFACTS
Motion Artifact

Physics

Motion artifacts in CT imaging can be caused by voluntary or involuntary patient movement such as swallowing during the scan acquisition. Patient motions commonly have a component occurring within the plane of image acquisition reconstruction (x,y). Thus, motion artifacts can severely impact those axial datasets most commonly viewed in CT imaging.[1] Movement of patient anatomies within a single field of view during a singular tube rotation time will ultimately cause the misregistration of the anatomy in the final image. Anatomies will be recorded in one physical location at one angle of rotation and another physical location at a differing angle of rotation. The appearance of anatomy in multiple pixel locations will either give the image an overall blurred appearance or will present as streaks across the imaged field of

Funding sources: S. Sammet was funded by the U.S. National Institutes of Health National Institute of Neurological Disorders and Stroke grant R25NS080949, the National Cancer Institute Education and Career Development program R25 Cancer Nanotechnology in Imaging and Radiotherapy (R25CA132822), the University of Chicago Comprehensive Cancer Center, and the Cancer Research Foundation.
Department of Radiology, University of Chicago, 5841 S Maryland Avenue, Chicago, IL 60637, USA
* Corresponding author.
E-mail address: dtg1@uchicago.edu

Neuroimag Clin N Am 32 (2022) 271–277
https://doi.org/10.1016/j.nic.2022.01.001
1052-5149/22/© 2022 Elsevier Inc. All rights reserved.

view (Fig. 1). This can result in abnormalities being obscured or simulated.

Solutions

- Avoid motion artifacts by having technologists coach patients about holding still during scans.
- Consider using a head holder to secure patients in place during scans. Make sure to inquire with the patient whether they are comfortable in their scan position.
- CT scanners offer features to over-scan a region beyond the standard 360° axial scan. This option will provide the reconstruction algorithm with additional views to potentially average out the presence of any unwanted anatomic motion.
- Reconstruct scans at multiple slice thicknesses, as it may be possible with thinner slices to isolate the motion to a smaller region with less diagnostic value or thicker slices may mask the artifact altogether.

Beam Hardening Artifact

Physics

Beam hardening artifacts are a direct result of x-ray attenuation properties resulting from the polychromatic energies of a CT beam. As a beam of x-ray photons transverses the tissues, the lower energy photons are preferentially attenuated (stopped within the body).[2] Beam travel through materials with high atomic numbers, that is, bone, metal, or CT contrast agents, intensify the removal of low energy photons. This process gradually leaves only photons of the highest

energy left in the beam to reach the detector. Tissue attenuation properties are a function of energy: as the overall energy of the beam increases, the attenuation coefficients decrease. This mechanism results in more photons on the exiting side of the beam, causing a darkening throughout the anatomic regions of lower atomic number. Typically, beam hardening artifacts will appear as a dark streak between 2 highly attenuating structures or a darkening in a central region surrounded by highly attenuating structures (Figs. 2 and 3). These artifacts are common in areas with highly attenuating structures, like bone.[3] The skull, particularly the posterior cranial fossa, is a common site for beam hardening artifacts.

Solutions

- Turn on beam hardening correction options. These corrections will use postprocessing to reduce the effects of beam hardening.[2]
- When scanning the neck, have the patient arms positioned on the side of the body rather than raised.
- Apply vendor-specific iterative reconstruction algorithms.[3]
- If beam hardening is making a clinical diagnosis difficult, consider scanning the patient in a dual-energy CT scanner. Dual-energy scanning provides the CT scanner and postprocessing algorithms information at 2 distinct x-ray photon energies, enabling the identification and subsequent elimination of beam hardening in the final reconstruction of images.[4,5]

Metal Streak Artifact

Physics

Metal artifacts consist of beam hardening, scatter, poisson noise (statistical error of low photon counts), photon starvation, and edge gradient effects.[6] This manifests as bright and dark bands radiating from metallic objects in the axial plane, which can potentially obscure surrounding tissues and lesions (Fig. 4). Some sources of metal streak artifact that can be encountered in the head and neck regions include dental amalgam and implants, cervical spine surgical hardware, bullet fragments, and eyelid weights.

Solutions

- Whenever possible, avoid scanning metallic objects in the imaging FOV.
- If it is known that metal exists along the path of the x-ray beam, consider increasing the energy of the scan (kV). This increase will

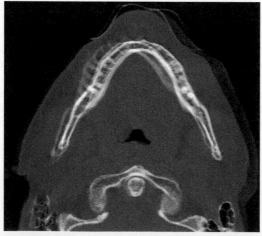

Fig. 1. Motion artifact. Axial CT images show apparent duplication and blurring of the osseous structures, potentially obscuring or mimicking fractures.

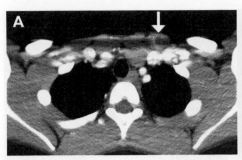

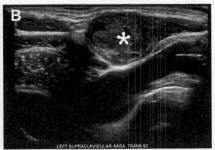

Fig. 2. Beam hardening artifact. Axial CT image (*A*) shows a left lower neck mass that is largely obscured by a dark band (*arrow*), but clearly visible on ultrasound (*) (*B*).

effectively preharden the beam, thereby decreasing the impact of the high atomic number metallic portion of the scan.

- Consider scanning the patient in a dual-energy CT scanner. Metal artifacts may be reduced on the virtual mono-energetic imaging generated from the dual-energy datasets.[7]
- Implement angled views to direct the streak artifact away from the area of interest (see **Fig. 4**).
- Apply vendor-specific metal artifact reduction algorithms (**Fig. 5**).[6]
- Consider scanning using a different imaging modality.

Windmill Artifact

Physics

Windmill artifact results from under-sampling along the z-axis during multislice helical CT scanning, whereby several rows of detectors intersect the plane of reconstruction during each rotation. In these instances, failure to interpolate data

properly between discrete detector locations produces alternating black and white patterns that resemble vanes of a windmill (**Fig. 6**).[3] This artifact occurs in areas with either steep or drastic Hounsfield unit (HU) differential anatomic changes along the z-axis, such as around the clavicles and through the base and top of the skull. The number of vanes increases with the pitch. While the artifact can obscure subtle imaging findings, it is readily recognized by its geometric and repeated configuration that does not resemble natural structures.

Solutions

- Implementing high-resolution reconstruction techniques or reconstructing thicker slices may minimize windmill artifacts.
- If rescanning is needed, consider lowering the scan pitch and reducing the rotation time. These adjustments should lessen the occurrence of these artifacts. They will ensure the table moves through the CT bore at a decreased speed, as the source rotates

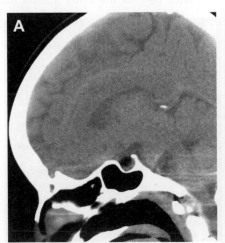

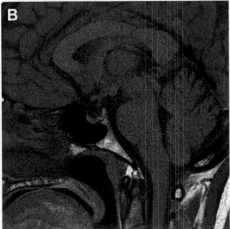

Fig. 3. Beam hardening artifact. Sagittal CT image (*A*) shows an area of apparent fat attenuation in the sella, which was interpreted as a possible dermoid or lipoma. Sagittal T_1-weighted head MR image of the pituitary gland performed shortly thereafter (*B*) shows no corresponding lesion in the sella turcica.

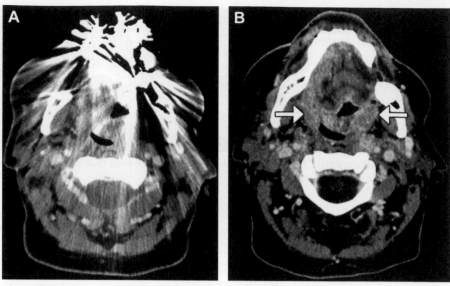

Fig. 4. Metal streak artifact and angled imaging. Standard axial CT image (*A*) shows extensive artifact from dental amalgam, which obscures an oropharyngeal tumor, the presence of the tumor (*arrows*) becomes evident on an angled scan that does not cover the dental filling (*B*).

around the patient at an increased speed, enabling a more thorough collection of information.[5]

Photon Starvation

Physics

Photon starvation artifacts are the result of an insufficient number of x-ray photons reaching the CT detector after passing through the patient.[2] The number of photons generated by the scanner is dependent on the tube current or mAs and should be adjusted according to the anatomy being imaged. Tube current modulation (TCM) techniques on most CT scanners are an example of a

technology developed to combat the occurrence of those projections with low photon counts during data acquisition which can lead to photon starvation in the final image. Excessive absorption of photons tends to occur in patients with large body habitus. The paucity of photons reaching the CT scanner detector results in a low signal-to-noise ratio, producing noisy images, known as quantum mottle (**Fig. 7**).

Solutions

- Ensure TCM and further organ dose modulation techniques (ie, "smart mA"), which modulates mA, as the x-ray source rotates 360°

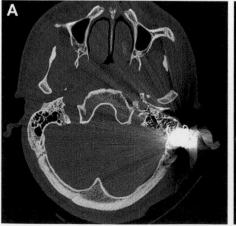
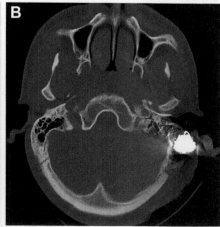

Fig. 5. Metal streak artifact and metal artifact reduction. Axial CT images of a patient with an embolization coil mass without (*A*) and with the implementation of metal artifact reduction software (*B*) demonstrate the effect of the streak artifact reduction after applying the software.

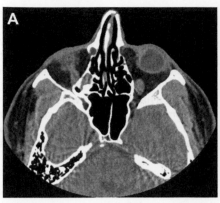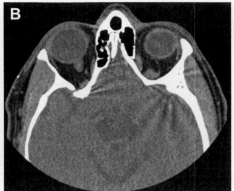

Fig. 6. Windmill artifacts. Axial maxillofacial CT images (*A*, *B*) show alternating bands of bright and dark radiating from sharp interfaces between bone and soft tissue.

around the patient, are enabled. These technologies allow the CT system to increase the photon output and decrease the likelihood of a detector element receiving too little signal to reconstruct the image.

- Vendor-specific reconstruction algorithms are offered to complete interpolation for regions surrounding a photon starvation artifact as an additional option for the postprocessing removal of this artifact.[2]
- Iterative reconstruction algorithms can mitigate the effects of photon starvation.[8]
- If the problem is persistent, then scanning the patient using a different imaging modality may be necessary.

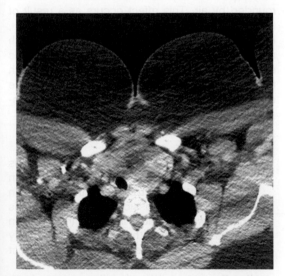

Fig. 7. Photon starvation. The axial CT image of the lower neck in a patient with a large body habitus is very noisy throughout.

Under-Sampling, Stair-Step, or Zebra Artifact

Physics
Under-sampling, stair-step, or zebra artifacts (**Fig. 8**) occur in CT imaging when the beam collimation is opened too wide or when using large reconstruction intervals.[2] Large reconstruction intervals lead to large spaces between adjacent image slices, which when reconstructed and placed side-by-side, display large changes over small distances. Merging these slices leads to discontinuities in the image that can appear as serrated edges or periodic horizontal stripes on sagittal and coronal reformatted images (see **Fig. 8**). The under-sampling effect is most conspicuous at the periphery of the images, as noise inhomogeneity is greatest off-axis, and can potentially mimic sin lacerations and fractures, for example.[2]

Solutions

- Refer to the source images in the axial plane.
- Reconstruct the images with "thinner" slices or overlapping sections, allowing the data to interpolate more effectively and resulting in a smoother transition between slices.[2]
- Use helical scanning or adaptive multiple plane reconstruction, which uses tilted planes for reconstruction, on CT scanners having this issue.

Ring Artifact

Physics
Ring artifacts (**Fig. 9**) result from broken or miscalibrated detector elements in multi-detector CT scanners.[2,8] Detector elements complete 360° of data collection around the bore of the CT scanner. When one detector element is not functioning, data dropout will appear in a full circle at a discrete radius. In helical mode, these artifacts can be

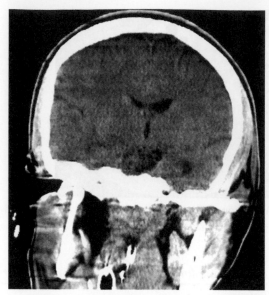

Fig. 8. Zebra artifact. Coronal image reconstructed from axial 5 mm thick slices obtained on a portable CT scanner shows multiple horizontal discontinuities at regular intervals.

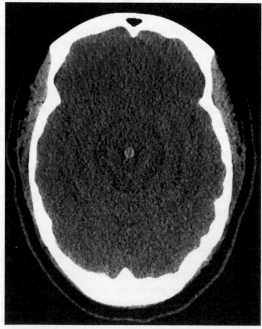

Fig. 9. Ring artifact. Axial head CT image shows a small bright ring in the center region of the FOV surrounded by several concentric dark rings.

difficult to spot as a single detector element is never responsible for the final image. However, when axial scans are taken at a slice width equal to the detector pixel width, ring artifacts become obvious presenting as discrete concentric rings of signal dropout (see **Fig. 9**). These are best visualized on a narrow window setting within a uniform phantom. If CT images are acquired with thicker slices, a dark concentric circle can appear from the averaging of slices with and without signal.

Solutions

- Recalibration of the detector elements should be completed.
- Reconstruct the CT images with thicker slices or image exclusively in helical scan modes. This will decrease the contributions of a single detector channel.
- If the issue persists after the detector is recalibrated, then a detector element in the CT array is a defect and needs to be replaced and a service engineer needs to be called.

Partial Volume Averaging Effects

Physics
Partial volume averaging artifacts in CT imaging occur in regions of nonuniform tissue. They are caused by an averaging of the different tissue attenuation properties contained within a single pixel that lead to the defining of an averaged HU for that pixel.[2] This can result in nonvisualization of small structures, such as the tympanic membrane and stapes. Or alternatively, regions of highly attenuating structures, such as the ossicles, may report lower than expected HU when surrounded by air. This effect occurs as a result of the HU no longer representing one single material, but rather an average of multiple materials, such as air and bone. Furthermore, certain structures can project beyond their actual margins and with the mixed attenuation can have the appearance of distinct lesions, particularly in the skull base region (**Fig. 10**).

Solutions

- If the imaging and reconstruction is completed at a slice thickness larger than the smallest pixel size, reconstruct the scan to the smallest possible option. While this change will inevitably increase the noise in the image, it offers the opportunity to clarify any regions of concern, should you suspect an impact from partial volume.[5]
- Iterative correction algorithms have been developed to address partial volume artifacts in helical scans.

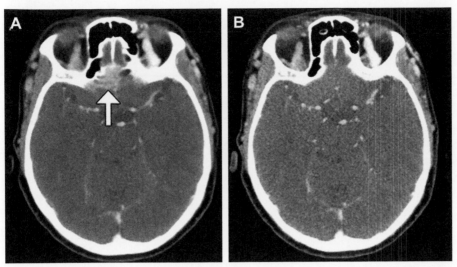

Fig. 10. Partial volume effects. Axial CT image reformatted with 3 mm slice thickness (*A*) shows an apparent area of hyper attenuation projecting along the anterior cranial fossa due to partial volume averaging with the underlying skull base, potentially mimicking a lesion, such as a meningioma. The artifact is no longer apparent on the axial CT image reformatted with a 1 mm slice thickness at the same level (*B*).

SUMMARY

Artifacts in medical imaging are not an infrequent occurrence. In some instances, their presence may obstruct anatomy, complicating the read of an image making a diagnosis difficult. On other occasions, they may instead provide valuable insight into the properties of objects within the imaging field of view. Understanding the basic principles of CT imaging will allow clinicians to interpret artifacts and weigh their significance. As the scope of CT imaging continues to broaden with multi-energy imaging, photon-counting detection, and implementation of advanced image processing algorithms, the resources available to mitigate and minimize patient and system CT artifacts will continue to expand. Continuing education and efforts toward understanding these tools will ensure guidance of an optimal CT imaging practice for patients and physicians alike.

CLINICS CARE POINTS

- Artifacts in head and neck CT imaging occur based on a variety of difference factors (patient, system, or reconstruction).

- Understanding the source of CT artifacts will allow mitigation strategies and/or diagnosis in spite of their presence.

- New technologies (wider beams, metal artifact reduction algorithms, dual-energy CT, ect) will continue building future solutions to artifacts.

DISCLOSURE

E. Marshall serves as a scientific consultant to Bayer HealthCare LLC. S. Sammet and D.T. Ginat have nothing to disclose.

REFERENCES

1. Yu H, Wang G. Data consistency based rigid motion artifact reduction in fan-beam CT. IEEE Trans Med Imaging 2007;26(2):249–60.

2. Barrett JF, Keat N. Artifacts in CT: recognition and avoidance. Radiographics 2004;24:1679–91.

3. Boas EF, Fleischmann D. CT artifacts: causes and reduction techniques. Imaging Med 2012;4(2):229–40.

4. Liao E, Srinivasan A. Applications of dual-energy computed tomography for artifact reduction in the head, neck, and spine. Neuroimaging Clin N Am 2017;27(3):489–97.

5. Gupta R. Neuro CT – What's a Good Head Exam? Technology Assessment Institute: Summit on CT Dose. 2011.

6. Kohan AA, Rubbert C, Vercher-Conejero JL, et al. The impact of orthopedic metal artifact reduction software on interreader variability when delineating areas of interest in the head and neck. Pract Radiat Oncol 2015;5(4):e309–15.

7. Roele ED, Timmer VCML, Vaassen LAA, et al. Dual-energy CT in head and neck imaging. Curr Radiol Rep 2017;5(5):19.

8. Ginat DT, Gupta R. Advances in computed tomography imaging technology. Annu Rev Biomed Eng 2014;16:431–53.

MR Imaging Artifacts in the Head and Neck Region
Pitfalls and Solutions

Emily L. Marshall, PhD, Daniel T. Ginat, MD, MS*, Steffen Sammet, MD, PhD

KEYWORDS

• MR imaging • Artifacts • Head and neck

KEY POINTS

- Artifacts in MR imaging can degrade image quality making diagnoses difficult.
- The underlying causes of individual MR imaging artifacts are identified and discussed.
- Possible solutions to eliminate each MR imaging artifact discussed are provided.
- Exposure to artifact examples and the underlying physics principles which generate these artifacts enable readers to assess clinical image artifacts in their daily practice.

Abbreviations	
MR	Magnetic Resonance

INTRODUCTION

MR imaging artifacts are aberrations that usually degrade image quality of MR images, but occasionally provide insights regarding actual imaging findings. The presence of artifacts can be attributed to various sources, including patient, scanner, and postprocessing factors. Artifacts can lead to diagnostic errors by obscuring findings or by being misinterpreted as lesions themselves. This article reviews various types of MR imaging artifacts that may be encountered during imaging of the head and neck region, beginning with explanations of the root cause of the artifact and ending with possible mitigation strategies. MR imaging systems are complex, so while the occurrence of artifacts cannot fully be eliminated, an awareness of their cause provides medical image reading physicians the tools to detect and read through their presence.

MR IMAGING ARTIFACTS
Motion Artifacts

Physics

Motion artifacts can be attributable to gross body movement or various involuntary organ movements, such as blood flow, swallowing, and respiration. Signal collection in the phase-encoding direction requires collection times on the order of tens of seconds. When anatomy shifts from one location to another during the phase-encoding signal collection period, the signal becomes assigned to the newly shifted location, and now misaligns to the earlier collected signal at the previous location. The extended period of data collection in MR imaging makes it particularly susceptible to patient motion. Frequently, patient motion artifacts appear as duplication and blurring of anatomic structures within a plane, but with a slight decrease in signal intensity (Fig. 1). Pulsatile flow artifacts, an involuntary form

Funding sources: S. Sammet was funded by the U.S. National Institutes of Health National Institute of Neurologic Disorders and Stroke grant R25NS080949, the National Cancer Institute Education and Career Development program R25 Cancer Nanotechnology in Imaging and Radiotherapy (R25CA132822), the University of Chicago Comprehensive Cancer Center, and the Cancer Research Foundation.
Department of Radiology, University of Chicago, 5841 S Maryland Avenue, Chicago, IL 60637, USA
* Corresponding author.
E-mail address: dtg1@uchicago.edu

Neuroimag Clin N Am 32 (2022) 279–286
https://doi.org/10.1016/j.nic.2022.01.002

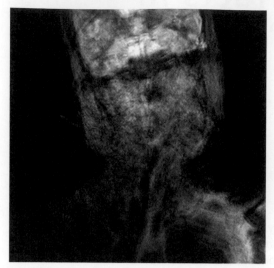

Fig. 1. Patient motion artifact. Coronal STIR (Short Tau Inversion Recovery) MR imaging of the neck shows extensive blurring with noise texture across the image, which degrades anatomic delineation.

of motion, are generated when blood flows through a slice and absorbs energy from the radiofrequency (RF) excitation pulse, but then continues to flow out of the slice before the signal readout and image formation.[1,2] The fresh blood that flows into the slice during signal readout comes from outside the desired slice and has not absorbed any RF energy and thus emits no signal during readout, appearing in the image as a black void (Fig. 2). In multislice sequences, blood experiencing an excitation pulse in one slice can flow into a neighboring slice and contribute to its signal.[3] The vessel lumen will then appear in a high signal intensity.

Solutions

- Consider swapping phase-encoding and frequency-encoding directions in an image.

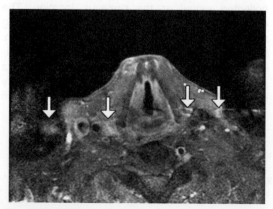

Fig. 2. Pulsation artifact. Axial postcontrast T1-weighted MR imaging shows vascular ghosts along the phase encoding direction (arrows).

Place the frequency-encoding direction along the dimension you want to best visualize.[1]
- If the motion is voluntary, consider using some type of immobilization device or scanning under sedation or general anesthesia.[2]
- Respiratory motion can be reduced or eliminated by breath-hold and respiratory trigger techniques to synchronize the data readout with the respiratory cycle of the patient.
- If motion is involuntary, application of anatomic gating techniques to match cardiac phases enables the MR imaging system to predict blood flow and align data collection to the cardiac cycle of the patient. Gating techniques are often complex and require adequate training of MR technologists.
- Decreasing the echo time (TE) provides the fastest solution to this problem. With the reduction of TE, data collection is occurring over a shortened period, and thus movement is less likely.[1]
- Suppression of blood signal via saturation bands can help to decrease the presence of flow artifacts as well.[2]

Susceptibility Artifact

Physics

The static magnetic field B_0 of an MR imaging scanner creates a magnetic moment by aligning protons in the patient's body within this magnetic field. Most tissues are diamagnetic, meaning they have no inherent magnetic moment until placed within a magnetic field, at which point they weakly oppose the magnetic field.[1] Paramagnetic and ferromagnetic materials, however, act differently and are attracted by magnetic fields by aligning with magnetic field lines.[3] Especially ferromagnetic materials experience strong attractive forces in a magnetic field and cause severe magnetic field distortions. The local distortion of the magnetic field by metallic objects changes the protons' precession frequencies in the human body leading to a misregistration of signal output to signal location.[2] Susceptibility artifacts typically appear as areas of signal void and distortion, which can obscure abnormalities (Fig. 3).

Solutions

- Remove the offending metallic object, if possible.
- The scan should be completed on a lower field strength magnet if an MR imaging compatible metallic implant or device is identified before the scan. Higher field strength magnets produce more severe susceptibility artifacts.

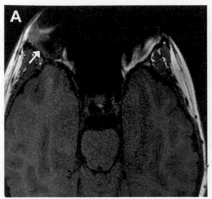
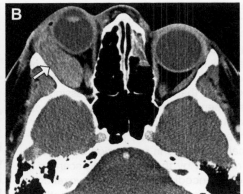

Fig. 3. Susceptibility artifact. Axial T1-weighted MR imaging (*A*) shows a right orbit mass (*arrow*) that is largely obscured by signal void from dental braces. The corresponding axial CT image (*B*) clearly depicts the right orbital tumor (*arrow*).

- Spin-echo–based protocols are recommended over gradient-echo–based protocols when scanning patients with implants.[1]
- Use a higher matrix and thinner slices.[4]
- Metal artifact reduction sequences can also help to reduce metal-induced susceptibility artifacts.
- Consider using another less artifact-prone imaging modality.

Partial Volume Artifact

Physics
Partial volume artifacts occur when tissue types with different resonance frequencies are imaged in the same image voxel. In such cases, that voxel will display in the final image with an intensity equivalent to the average of the tissues within it. The signal within that individual voxel becomes difficult to interpret, as it no longer reflects details of separate anatomic structures, but instead consists of an average of signals.[3] Ultimately, a partial volume artifact is a form of undersampling, in which the matrix size is inappropriately low for the selected field of view (FOV), or the slice

thickness is too large. This results in blurred images that can be difficult to interpret (**Fig. 4**) and in which small lesions might be missed. When high-resolution images are needed in MR, it is important to consider both in-plane (conventionally speaking x-y resolution) and through-plane (conventionally z resolution) resolutions.[3] As spatial resolution is improved, noise in the final images will increase, understanding this relationship and selecting the resolution relevant to diagnosis is essential.

Solutions

- Decrease the pixel size with same field of view to increase matrix size.[3]
- Decrease the slice thickness.

Chemical Shift Artifact

Physics
Chemical shift artifact can occur as a result of the precession frequency differences of the protons, dependent upon their immediate surroundings. MR imaging relies on the characterization of the

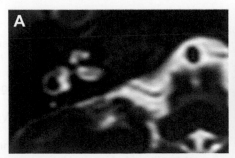
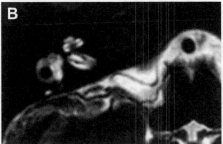

Fig. 4. Partial volume artifact. Axial DRIVE (driven equilibrium radio frequency reset pulse) MR imaging obtained with a matrix of 156 × 104 shows blurry anatomy, in which cochlear nerve deficiency could not be excluded (*A*). The repeat axial DRIVE MR imaging obtained with a matrix of 300 × 298, with otherwise identical field of view, shows a sharper delineation of the anatomy in the inner ear (*B*), with an intact cochlear nerve.

proton resonance frequencies and makes use of this information to localize the signals.[5] Small shifts in proton precession frequencies occur based on the chemical compound and accompanying chemical bonds that the proton is a part of. The hydrogen protons in fat precess at a slightly lower frequency than water (this precession frequency is dependent on the strength of the main magnet, at 1.5 T the precession frequency difference between water and fat is about 220 Hz).[6] These small deviations in precession frequencies are then read out by the MR imaging scanner in the frequency encoding direction. If a voxel contains both water and fat protons, and is read out at the water frequency, the signal from fat protons will appear to come from water protons in a lower part of the field and the location of the fat protons will be spatially mismapped. This leads to signal shifts in corresponding voxels in the frequency encoding direction.[7] The chemical shift artifact appears as dark or light bands at the interfaces of tissues with different chemical compositions (Fig. 5), which can potentially mimic hemorrhage, for example.[2]

Solutions

- An increase in receiver bandwidth can decrease the thickness of the chemical shift ribbon-like artifact. This action increases the frequencies collected per pixel, shrinking the width in pixels of the artifact.[3]
- Optimize fat-suppression sequences on your MR imaging scanner. Removal of the fat signal from the images, using techniques like fat-saturation pulses, makes chemical shift artifacts disappear.[6]

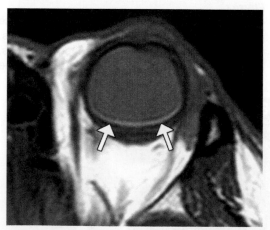

Fig. 5. Chemical shift artifact. Axial T1-weighted MR imaging shows silicone oil in the left globe with an artifactual rim of high signal along posterior aspect of the oil in the frequency encoding direction (*arrows*).

- Increase in static magnetic field strength increases the differences between fat and water precession frequencies, making these artifacts more apparent at higher field strengths. Consider scanning with a lower field strength MR imaging system.[7]

Fat Suppression Failure

Physics

Fat suppression artifacts result from small differences in the precession frequency of fat and water protons.[5] The small resonance frequency difference of fat and water protons can be exploited to cancel specific signals from fat protons out of the final image through fat-saturation, inversion recovery, or opposed phase imaging techniques.[1] Fat-saturation techniques apply an RF pulse, tuned to exactly match the fat precession frequency, before the imaging sequence. This fat-selective RF pulse is immediately followed by a spoiler gradient to dephase the fat signals, making it impossible for the fat protons to rephase, a step needed in MR imaging to produce a signal. The fat-saturation preparation is followed by the desired imaging sequence, resulting in signal collection from nonfat molecules such as water molecules. The result is an image with fat darkened. Failures in fat saturation create an appearance of nondistinct bright areas that can potentially mimic enhancement of post-contrast T1-weighted sequences and often occur in the supraclavicular regions (Fig. 6). The fat-saturation technique relies on the very small difference in fat and water precession frequencies and any shifts in these expected values will lead to non-uniformities. Inversion-recovery techniques for fat suppression are based on differences in the T1 relaxation time of tissues. T1 of fat tissue is shorter than T1 of water. After a 180° inversion pulse, the longitudinal magnetization of fat will recover faster than that of water. If an excitation pulse is then applied at the null point of fat tissue, fat will produce no signal, whereas water will still produce a signal.

Solutions

- If you intend to use fat-suppression techniques, use an active shimming technique before the scan. This will improve the magnetic field homogeneity making image nonuniformities less likely.[8]
- When possible, use a smaller FOV to avoid magnetic inhomogeneities.
- Scan the patient on a magnet with higher field strength. At higher static magnetic field strengths, B_0, the differences in precession frequencies of fat and water increase, making these techniques easier to implement.[1]

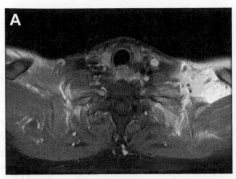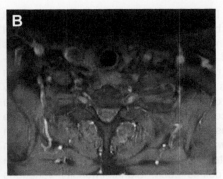

Fig. 6. Axial fat-saturated postcontrast T1-weighted MR imaging shows incomplete elimination of fat signal in the left supraclavicular fossa region (A). Axial postcontrast T1-weighted MR imaging obtained using mDixon fat suppression technique with smaller field of view shows complete elimination of fat signal (B).

- Try opposed phase or Dixon fat-suppression techniques, which provide more reliable results (see Fig. 6).[7]
- If the fat-suppression techniques continue to fail, call a service engineer to correct the passive shim of the MR imaging system.

Wrap-around or Aliasing Artifact.

Physics
Phase encoding gradients are applied across the entire body, not just the anatomy of interest or designated FOV. When a FOV is selected on the localizer scan, a small portion of the gradient is selected to contribute to the image. In addition, distinguishable phase changes of protons are limited to the 360° of a circle. This becomes obvious when considering that the angles of +90° and −270° are equivalent when drawn onto a circle. To capture finite differences in the samples' proton phases, the sampling rate must be 2 times the maximum frequency of the object.[9] This limiting sample rate represents the Nyquist frequency.[1] Aliasing is a phenomenon in signal processing that occurs when signals become indistinguishable (or aliases of one another) when sampled below the Nyquist frequency. Wrap-around or aliasing artifacts occur in MR imaging when the protons within anatomy outside of the imaged FOV precessing at a higher rate are improperly assigned to mismapped phase shifts during image data interpretation making them appear equivalent to others within the imaged FOV (Fig. 7). This would arise when anatomy outside the FOV with proton phase shifts of −270° wraps up and around onto the opposing side of the image, where proton phase shifts of +90° were included in the FOV and are displayed in the image.

Solutions

- Increase the FOV when planning the imaging series on the scout images, to maintain spatial resolution increase the number of phase encoding steps accordingly. If all anatomy is included in the FOV then all proton phase shifts will be unique, lying between −180° and +180°.[2]
- Apply the phase encoding direction to the smaller anatomic dimension, for example, through the chest use the phase encoding in the patient's anterior-posterior direction as opposed to the lateral direction.[9]
- Make use of the machine setting fold-over suppression/phase oversampling, but in most cases these settings require more than one average, leading to longer scan times.[3]

Signal Intensity Artifacts

Physics
Signal intensity artifacts are variations of the signal intensity in an MR imaging that are not related to the intrinsic characteristics of the tissues being

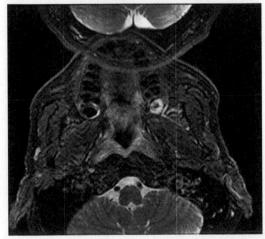

Fig. 7. Wrap-around artifact. Axial T2-weighted MR imaging shows that the posterior portion of the head projects onto the anterior part of the head.

imaged. These artifacts are inherent in surface coil imaging but can also be caused by improper coil positioning or system malfunction. Surface coils are used in MR imaging to improve image signal-to-noise ratios, whereby the detection of the small signals is highly dependent on geometric proximity to the protons.[9] The most desirable configuration of surface coils is therefore adjacent to the tissue of interest. The effects of such a configuration are shown in **Fig. 8**, where a steep decrease in signal intensity with increasing distance from the surface coil is seen. Signal intensity variations can also occur due to a lack of protocol optimization. For example, signal changes can appear in MR imaging when suppression pulses are inadequately applied, leaving behind signals in undesirable regions. These undesired signals can then be amplified by the coil sensitivity profile, presenting as a gray tint throughout the region. The appearance of regional signal variations can also be the result of coil malfunction or a broken receiver element within a multielement coil.

Solutions

- Proper patient and coil positioning is an easy remedy for positioning-related signal intensity variations in MR images.
- Protocol optimization and proper positioning of saturation bands.
- If a coil element has failed, the coil must be replaced by the unit vendor. Image quality will suffer until the coil is replaced.

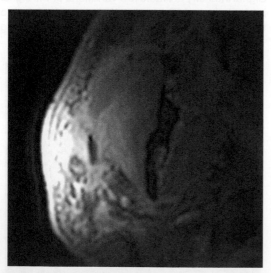

Fig. 8. Signal intensity artifact. Axial postcontrast T1-weighted MR imaging of the right face obtained using a surface microscopy coil shows a much higher signal in the superficial tissues near the coil than in the deeper tissues.

B_1-inhomogeneity Artifact

Physics

Although the main magnetic field, B_0, aligns proton spins, the RF field, B_1, tilts proton spins and alters their alignment with B_0. B_1-fields are emitted at the Larmor frequency, a property that defines the precession frequency of protons about B_0. Once the RF pulse is turned off, the protons will relax back into their steady-state aligned with B_0. The protons emit energy as they relax back to their steady-state, which induces currents in the receiver coil and subsequently produces the MR image. RF pulses are typically generated within the large bore of the MR system by the body transmitter at a considerable distance from the patient. Small differences in the applied RF pulse across a FOV will result in some protons receiving more energy compared with others.[1] This difference in absorbed energy will produce a nonuniform image (**Fig. 9**).[8] Inhomogeneities in the B_1-field most frequently manifest as bright and dark regions in the patient image; sometimes these fluctuations in intensity can be even seen within the same tissue.

Solutions

- Scan the patient in a scanner with a lower static magnetic field strength B_0. High and ultrahigh

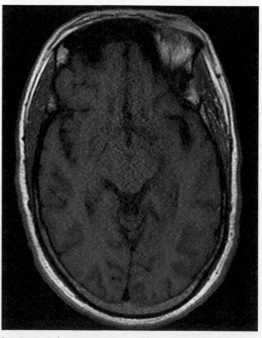

Fig. 9. B_1-inhomogeneity artifact. Axial T1-weighted MR imaging shows higher levels of noise in the central part of the images.

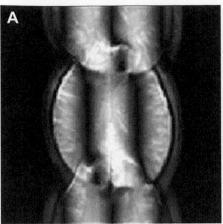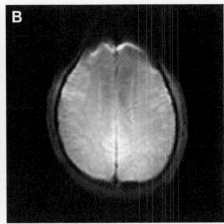

Fig. 10. Eddy current artifact. Axial MR images show a scan completed without enabling eddy current compensation techniques (*A*) and the same scan once eddy current compensation was enabled (*B*). (*Courtesy* of GE Healthcare, Waukesha, WI.)

field MR imaging scanners experience, in general, more severe B_1-inhomogeneities.[1]

- Apply B_1-mapping and B_1-inhomogeneity correction.[8]
- Call the service engineer on-site to optimize the B_1-field shimming. The applied B_1-field, much like the B_0-field, can also be shimmed for higher homogeneity.[1]

Eddy Current

Physics

MR imaging systems follow Faraday's law, which states that changes in magnetic field induce a voltage V, and current I, according to Ohm's law:

$$V = I \bullet R$$

where R is the resistance of the conductor. During image acquisition, swift changes in RF pulses and magnetic gradients induce regional currents in tissue.[1] These currents negatively impact the homogeneity of the main magnetic field B_0, resulting in imaging distortion. Alterations in the main magnetic field influence the final image in multiple ways, including blurring, stretching, textural changes, image repetition, and ghosting (**Fig. 10**). Newer MR imaging systems use a combination of active gradient shielding, to counteract current induction, and image postprocessing to decrease the impact of eddy currents on the final image.

Solutions

- Use slower scanning protocols (non-EPI).[10]
- Guarantee application of eddy current reduction algorithms during postprocessing.
- Call the service engineer on-site to calibrate the system to ensure full engagement of eddy current compensation techniques.[1]

Data Error Artifact

Physics

K-space mapping, frequency versus phase, directly dictates image formation in MR imaging. This unique intermediary step has a tendency to amplify hardware issues. Data error artifacts are a result of poor receiver electronics, faulty internal connections or external signals that lead to a single bright point in k-space receiving an erroneously large signal, also known as k-space spike artifact.[9] Because every single point in k-space contains imaged data for all pixels in the reconstructed image, this single point makes a large impact. The artifact presents across the entire MR image, as a repeating set of parallel lines at a certain spatial frequency (**Fig. 11**). The

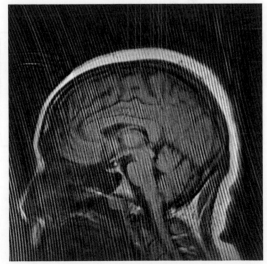

Fig. 11. Data error k-space spike artifact. Sagittal T1-weighted MR imaging shows repeating bands of alternating dark and bright signal intensities across the image.

location of the spike in k-space determines the density, as well as the angulation of the lines across the resulting MR image.

Solutions

- Reprocessing the raw data may remove this artifact.
- Attempt to scan a phantom with a different receiver coil to assess whether the issue originates from the coil. If the problem resolves after changing the coil, the scanner can continue to operate and the faulty coil needs to be removed from clinical use.
- If troubleshooting fails and the issue is determined to reside within the MR imaging system, the field service engineer must be contacted to service the MR imaging scanner.

SUMMARY

MR imaging artifacts are features appearing in MR images that are not present in the original anatomy. MR imaging artifacts can be patient-related, hardware-related, or signal-processing–related and affect diagnostic quality or mimic pathology. It is necessary to take MR imaging artifacts into consideration when interpreting images. A basic knowledge of MR imaging physics and the potential origin of MR imaging artifacts can help to find solutions to eliminate or reduce the influence of artifacts on image quality by adjusting acquisition parameters appropriately for a better diagnosis.

CLINICS CARE POINTS

- Understanding the origin and physics of MR imaging artifacts (patient-related, hardware-related, or signal-processing–related) is important when interpreting images and can help to improve image quality by reducing or eliminating these artifacts.

DISCLOSURE

E. Marshall serves as a scientific consultant to Bayer HealthCare LLC. S. Sammet and D. Ginat have nothing to disclose.

REFERENCES

1. Morelli JN, Runge VM, Ai F, et al. An image-based approach to understanding the physics of MR artifacts. Radiographics 2011;31(3):849–66.
2. Krupa K, Bekiesińska-Figatowska M. Artifacts in Magnetic Resonance Imaging. Polish J Radiol 2015;80:93–106.
3. McRobbie DW, Moore EA, Graves MG, et al. From Picture to proton. 3rd edition. Cambridge University Press; 2016. Chapters 2 and 7: pgs 18-21 and 81 - 101.
4. De Foer B, Vercruysse JP, Pilet B, et al. Single-shot, turbo spin-echo, diffusion-weighted imaging versus spin-echo-planar, diffusion-weighted imaging in the detection of acquired middle ear cholesteatoma. AJNR Am J Neuroradiol 2006;27(7):1480–2.
5. Eggers H, Börnert P. Chemical shift encoding-based water-fat separation methods. J Magn Reson Imaging 2014;40(2):251–68.
6. Imaizumi A, Yoshino N, Yamada I, et al. A potential pitfall of MR imaging for assessing mandibular invasion of squamous cell carcinoma in the oral cavity. Am J Neuroradiol 2006;27(1):114–22.
7. Ma J. Dixon techniques for water and fat imaging. J Magn Reson Imaging 2008;28(3):543–58.
8. Truong TK, Chakeres DW, Beversdorf DQ, et al. Effects of static and radiofrequency magnetic field inhomogeneity in ultra-high field magnetic resonance imaging. Magn Reson Imaging 2006;24(2):103–12.
9. Bushberg JT, Seibert JA, Leidholdt EM, et al. The essential physics of medical imaging. 3rd edition. Lippincott Williams & Wilkins; 2001. Chapter 13; pg 474 - 499.
10. Bammer R, Markl M, Barnett A, et al. Analysis and generalized correction of the effect of spatial gradient field distortions in diffusion-weighted imaging. Magn Reson Med 2003;50:560–9.

Pearls and Pitfalls of 18FDG-PET Head and Neck Imaging

Randy Yeh, MD[a], Ahmad Amer, BS[b], Jason Michael Johnson, MD[c], Daniel T. Ginat, MD, MS[d],*

KEYWORDS

• PET • False positive • False negative • Head • Neck

KEY POINTS

- Certain artifacts and normal activity in the head and neck can potentially mimic lesions on FDG-PET/CT studies.
- As FDG is not specific only to malignancy, it can accumulate in a variety of benign processes including benign tumors, inflammatory, posttreatment conditions.
- Conversely, certain head and neck cancers are not particularly FDG avid and can lead to false-negative interpretations.
- Lesion characterization on anatomic imaging is complementary to PET.

INTRODUCTION

The management of head and neck cancer is a multidisciplinary effort often involving oncologic surgery, plastic and reconstructive surgery, radiation therapy, chemotherapy, and immunotherapy. Complicated and variable approaches to surgical resection, local tissue reconstruction, neck dissection, radiation therapy and induction, concurrent and neoadjuvant chemotherapy/immunotherapy regimens can complicate imaging findings during and after treatment.[1,2]

Diagnostic imaging plays an important role in the treatment of head and neck cancer. The critical phases of diagnostic imaging begin with accurate initial local staging and exclusion of distant metastatic disease. Thus, accurately assessing whether upstaging tumor features are present that may suggest an alternative treatment pathway; accurate cervical nodal staging along with the identification of involvement of nodal station and laterality; and

assessment for distant metastatic disease.[3] There are many radiotracers available, but ^{18}F-fluorodeoxyglucose (FDG) is the most commonly used due to its widespread availability, relatively low cost, and accuracy.[4] [18]FDG-PET/CT (positron emission tomography/computed tomography) plays a major role in the initial staging of head and neck cancer.[2,4,5] It also facilitates the appropriate management of patients with head and neck cancer in whom treatment is expensive and associated with a significant morbidity.[5,6]

There are many potential pitfalls associated with [18]FDG-PET/CT imaging. The purpose of this article is to review the most common interpretation pitfalls related to head and neck PET/CT and how to avoid them.

TECHNICAL ISSUES

Artifacts related to metallic implants. Permanent dental hardware and metallic implants can

[a] Department of Radiology, Molecular Imaging and Therapy Service, Memorial Sloan Kettering Cancer Center, 1275 York Avenue, New York, NY 10065, USA; [b] Department of Neuroradiology, The University of Texas MD Anderson Cancer Center, MSIII, Chicago Medical School at Rosalind Franklin University of Medicine and Science, 1500 Holcombe Boulevard, Houston, TX 77030, USA; [c] Department of Neuroradiology, The University of Texas MD Anderson Cancer Center, 1500 Holcombe Boulevard, Houston, TX 77030, USA; [d] Department of Radiology, University of Chicago, 5841 S Maryland Avenue, Chicago, IL 60637, USA
* Corresponding author.
E-mail address: dtg1@uchicago.edu

Neuroimag Clin N Am 32 (2022) 287–298
https://doi.org/10.1016/j.nic.2022.01.005

degrade the appearance of CT, PET, and MRI by causing streak artifacts and distortion of the magnetic field.[7,8] These artifacts tend to cause issues with PET interpretation through issues with CT-based attenuation correction factors, but metallic implants can also absorb the photons from F-18 decay and lead to issues with the PET image reconstruction (**Fig. 1**). Metal artifact reduction software can help improve the appearance of the CT image and inspection of the emission scan series (nonattenuation-corrected) helps clarify uncertainty regarding the presence of CT-based attenuation artifact.[9,10]

Misregistration. [18]FDG-PET/CT is more accurate than [18]FDG-PET alone in the identification and localization of head and neck cancer which aids in appropriate staging and treatment planning.[11–15] However, automated software methods for coregistered PET and CT data are prone to errors most commonly related to patient motion between sequentially acquired data sets.[16] Misregistration refers to superimposing areas of activity on the incorrect anatomic structures seen on CT. It is typically caused by different patient positioning between the PET and CT scans (**Fig. 2**).[17] This issue can lead to both false-negative and false-positive findings as the PET activity is projected onto the wrong structure. Eliminating or reducing the time interval between PET and CT acquisition can be immensely beneficial for avoiding misregistration.[16] Misregistration can also be corrected manually or with software coregistration when necessary.[16]

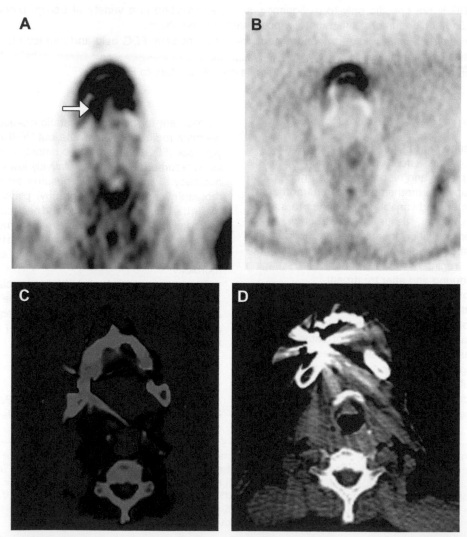

Fig. 1. Attenuation correction artifact. Attenuation corrected (*A*), nonattenuation corrected (*B*), fused [18]FDG-PET-CT (*C*), and CT (*D*) show an erroneous focus of hypermetabolism adjacent to a dental implant, as the [18]FDG avid focus is not present on the uncorrected image.

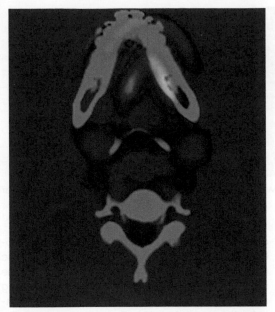

Fig. 2. Misregistration. The 18FDG-PET and CT images are not properly aligned, such that the left sublingual gland activity projects over the mandible.

NORMAL PHYSIOLOGIC ACTIVITY

Normal anatomic structures can display varying degrees of uptake on 18FDG-PET (**Table 1**).

Brown fat. In response to sympathetic stimulation, brown fat over-expresses glucose transporter 4 (GLUT4), resulting in an influx of glucose and foci of 18FDG avidity on PET/CT.[22] While initially thought to only be present in newborns, PET/CT has revealed that brown fat can persist into adulthood.[23] Brown fat is most often present in the supraclavicular and posterior neck regions (**Fig. 3**) and is particularly active in cold environments. Brown fat is most often symmetric, but is occasionally asymmetric. When evaluating a patient for malignancy with PET/CT, brown fat and tumor can show similar uptake characteristics, and can therefore be easily confused.[23] In every case, the presence of brown fat should be confirmed with CT correlation showing corresponding areas of fat attenuation in the range of −50 to −150 HU, as opposed to soft tissue attenuation that would otherwise characterize hypermetabolic malignant lesions, such as lymph nodes (**Fig. 4**).[22] To reduce the 18FDG uptake of brown fat, it is helpful to keep the patient warm by using heating blankets and appropriately controlling the temperature of the room. Additionally, medications such as fentanyl, propranolol, or diazepam can be administered and the patient should be encouraged to follow a high-fat, low-carbohydrate diet before 18FDG injection.[23]

Muscles. Although patients are advised not to engage in strenuous physical activity or speaking before their 18FDG-PET examinations, elevated physiologic muscle activity is often encountered on 18FDG-PET and can potentially mimic tumors or inflammation. Common sites of physiologic muscle uptake in the neck include the paraspinal muscles secondary to strain, the masseter muscles from chewing, and the vocal cords from speaking (**Fig. 5**). The physiologic activity can be recognized by the fact that the hypermetabolism is confined to the boundaries of the muscles involved, often with a diffuse linear rather than focal configuration. The activity can be asymmetric, particularly after surgery and/or

Table 1 Typical SUV for head and neck tissues	
Normal Tissue	**Mean Standardized Uptake Value (SUV)[18–21]**
Blood	1.0
Bone Marrow	2.2
Brain Cortex	11.4
Cerebellum	7.2
Fat	0.3
Lymph nodes	1.6
Muscle	1.5
Salivary glands	sublingual (2.9), submandibular (2.1), parotid (1.9)
Tonsils	palatine (3.5), lingual (3.1)
Thyroid	1.3

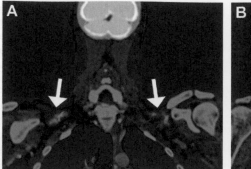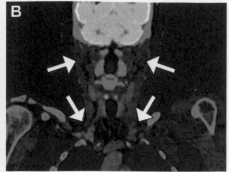

Fig. 3. Brown fat. Coronal fused [18]FDG-PET/CT images show prominent FDG avidity in the bilateral supraclavicular fossae and posterior triangles of the neck (*arrows*).

denervation, which can be somewhat confounding. However, comparison with anatomic imaging, such as CT or MRI, can help evaluate for the presence of an underlying lesion (**Fig. 6**).

Salivary Glands. Normal physiologic processes lead to [18]FDG accumulation in the salivary glands whereby it is secreted into saliva. Salivary gland activity on [18]FDG-PET can be variable, but often seems as bilaterally symmetric activity that is higher than background activity (**Fig. 7**).[24–29] Asymmetrical submandibular gland uptake can occur in patients who have undergone surgical removal of a gland with contralateral hypertrophy and in patients who have undergone unilateral radiation therapy.[27] Asymmetrical uptake, especially when focal and with a corresponding CT correlate, should warrant further radiological and histopathological correlation to rule out disease involvement.

Normal lymphoid tissues. [18]FDG uptake can be very pronounced in the Waldeyer ring tissues due to high cellular activity. This normal physiologic metabolic activity is typically symmetric (**Fig. 8**), but can be asymmetric especially in the setting of prior surgery and radiation. The imaging appearance alone is typically sufficient to differentiate the normal metabolic appearance of the pharyngeal lymphoid tissue, but cases of extranodal lymphoma and squamous cell carcinoma of the nasopharynx or base of the tongue may be bilateral.[30]

FALSE-POSITIVE CONDITIONS

Vocal cord palsy. Asymmetric [18]FDG uptake in the vocal cords can also be mistaken for malignancy in patients with laryngeal nerve palsy. The paralyzed vocal cord tends to be atrophic and devoid of metabolic activity, while the nonparalyzed vocal cord tends to compensate for its weakened counterpart, leading to increased metabolism and therefore [18]FDG uptake (**Fig. 9**). In addition, the

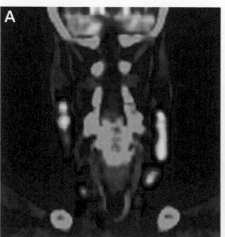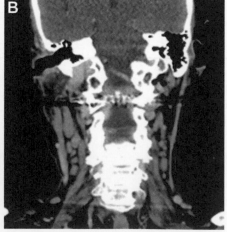

Fig. 4. Lymphoma. Coronal fused [18]FDG-PET/CT (*A*) and coronal CT (*B*) images show bilateral hypermetabolic cervical lymphadenopathy.

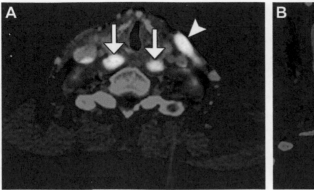
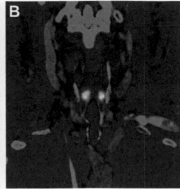

Fig. 5. Physiologic muscle activity. Axial 18FDG-PET/CT fusion image (*A*) shows diffuse activity in the bilateral longus colli muscles (*arrows*) and in the left sternocleidomastoid muscle (*arrowhead*). The patient had previously undergone right neck dissection. Coronal 18FDG-PET/CT fusion image in a different patient (*B*) shows activity in the bilateral vocal cords.

thyroarytenoid and posterior cricoarytenoid muscles can also appear as focal hypermetabolic areas on 18FDG-PET.[31]

Soft tissue infection and inflammation. Inflammation, infection, and granulomatous diseases can display increased 18FDG uptake, thereby mimicking malignancy (**Figs. 10–12**). Increased glycolysis in inflammatory cells, particularly macrophages, during infection leads to an increased uptake of 18FDG.[32] The acquisition of a baseline imaging examination is important to serve as a reference for evaluation in the posttreatment follow-up for patients with cancer. Surgery alters the normal anatomy, tissue planes, and landmarks in the head and neck.[32–35] Radiation treatment induces tissue edema, microvascular injury, and fibrosis. Chemotherapy can also lead to inflammatory changes within the head and neck whether due to tumor necrosis-related inflammation or subclinical infectious activity.[30] These posttreatment effects can be difficult to distinguish from tumor recurrence on PET (**Fig. 13**). Thus, the baseline imaging examination should be optimally performed at the time when most postoperative changes have resolved and when tumor recurrence rarely occurs.[30] A baseline examination with CT or MRI can be performed 8 to 10 weeks after treatment, while the initial 18FDG-PET scan is ideally performed approximately 12 weeks after the completion of radiation therapy.[36]

Reactive lymph nodes. While 18FDG-PET is highly sensitive for the detection of lymph node metastases, a major limitation is a lack of specificity. In particular, reactive lymphadenitis

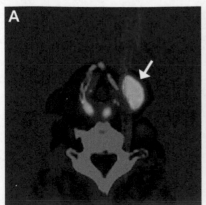
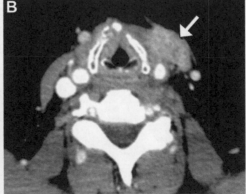

Fig. 6. Intramuscular metastasis. Axial fused 18FDG-PET/CT (*A*) and diagnostic CT (*B*) images show a hypermetabolic mass in the left sternocleidomastoid muscle, which represents tumor recurrence in a patient with a history of laryngeal cancer.

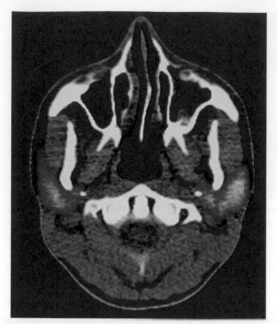

Fig. 7. Physiologic salivary gland activity. Axial ¹⁸FDG-PET/CT fusion image shows diffuse hypermetabolism in the bilateral parotid glands.

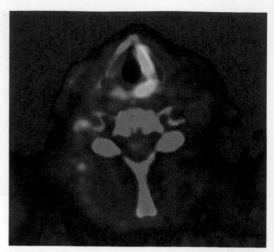

Fig. 9. Vocal cord palsy. Axial ¹⁸FDG-PET-CT shows asymmetric metabolic activity in the intact left vocal cord, but atrophy of the right vocal cord with the paucity of activity.

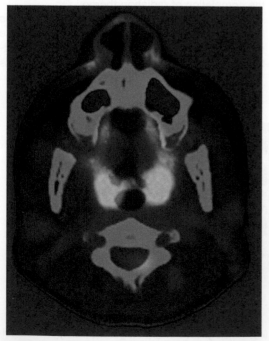

Fig. 8. Axial ¹⁸FDG-PET-CT image shows normal hypermetabolism in the bilateral tonsils in a young patient.

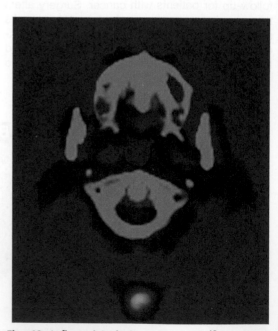

Fig. 10. Inflamed inclusion cyst. Axial ¹⁸FDG-PET-CT shows a hypermetabolic nodule in the posterior neck subcutaneous tissues.

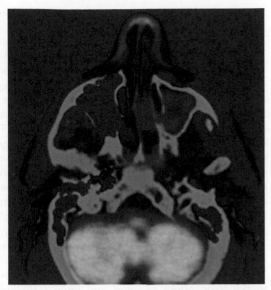

Fig. 11. Sinusitis. Axial 18FDG-PET/CT shows hypermetabolism associated with the inflamed mucosa in the left maxillary sinus.

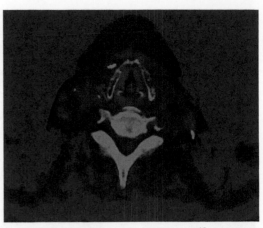

Fig. 13. Postoperative inflammation. 18FDG-PET/CT performed about 7 weeks after bilateral neck dissection shows diffuse soft tissue hypermetabolism.

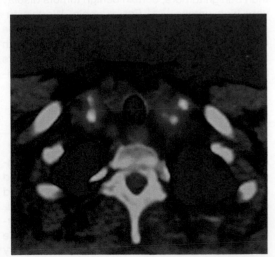

Fig. 12. Sarcoidosis. Axial 18FDG-PET/CT shows hypermetabolic lymph nodes in the neck bilaterally.

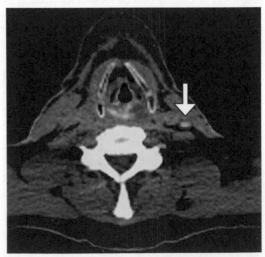

Fig. 14. Reactive lymph node. 18FDG-PET-CT image shows a small mildly hypermetabolic left level 3 lymph node (arrow) based on excisional biopsy in a patient previously treated for head and neck cancer.

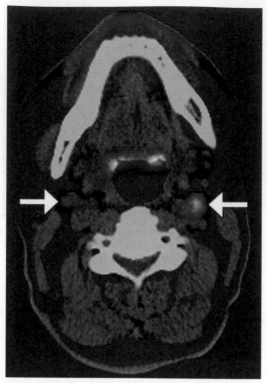

Fig. 15. Sarcoid-like reaction related to immunotherapy. Axial [18]FDG-PET/CT fusion image shows hypermetabolic lymph nodes in the neck bilaterally.

represents an inflammatory process that can occur in a variety of settings and can display elevated [18]FDG avidity. This phenomenon can be indistinguishable from neoplasm on [18]FDG-PET or based on size criteria (**Fig. 14**).[37] Ultimately, follow-up or biopsy can be helpful for making the distinction. The false-positive finding on [18]FDG-PET is attributable to follicular dendritic cells in

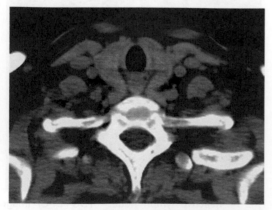

Fig. 16. Thyroiditis related to immunotherapy. Axial [18]FDG-PET/CT fusion image shows diffuse hypermetabolism in the thyroid gland.

the germinal centers of secondary lymph node follicles.[38]

Immunotherapy-related adverse effects. Immunotherapy can lead to potentially confounding findings on metabolic imaging related to either inflammatory responses or immune-related adverse events, including sarcoid-like reactions, thyroiditis, and myositis, for example, Each of these entities demonstrates hypermetabolism on [18]FDG-PET (**Figs. 15 and 16**). Furthermore, immunotherapy can lead to pseudoprogression, in which favorable treatment response can mimic disease progression on imaging. This phenomenon is attributable to the desired inflammatory response to the neoplasm and has been most commonly reported in cases of melanoma treated with anti-CTLA-4 therapy, whereby as many as 15% of patients experience pseudoprogression.[39]

Mucosal necrosis. Mucosal necrosis is a potential toxic effect of head and neck radiation therapy that tends to occur during the first 6 to 12 months after treatment.[40] [18]FDG-PET imaging can reveal hypermetabolism associated with areas of ulceration (**Fig. 17**), which can potentially mimic recurrence. On CT and MRI, mucosal necrosis shows a lack of mucosal enhancement with the breech of the mucosa. The presence of gas adjacent to the lesion is also suggestive of necrosis. However, if the ulceration is associated with adjacent soft tissue enhancement, the differentiation between radiation necrosis and recurrent tumor becomes difficult. Ultimately, mucosal complications are generally moreup easily diagnosed based on clinical examination than with imaging.

Benign neoplasms. Although malignant neoplasms generally display higher [18]FDG uptake than benign tumors, certain benign tumors display very high uptake.[41–44] For example, Warthin tumors are often located in the parotid tails, can be bilateral, and display high [18]FDG uptake with SUV indistinguishable from malignant tumors (**Fig. 18**).[45] Ultimately, a biopsy might be considered for more definite clarification.

FALSE-NEGATIVE CONDITIONS

Hypometabolic primary cancers. Certain malignant head and neck neoplasms, such as adenoid cystic carcinomas, low-grade mucoepidermoid carcinomas, necrotic primary squamous cell carcinomas, well-differentiated papillary thyroid cancer, and spindle cell carcinomas, may have little or no [18]FDG-avidity (**Fig. 19**).[30] Low-grade salivary gland cancers also have lower SUV than high grade malignancies.[30]

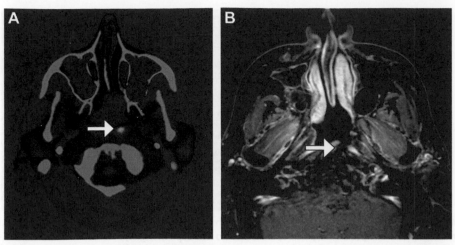

Fig. 17. Mucosal ulceration. Axial ¹⁸FDG-PET/CT (*A*) shows a small area of hypermetabolism along the posterior pharyngeal wall (*arrow*) with a corresponding nonenhancing defect (*arrow*) on the postcontrast axial fat-suppressed MRI (*B*).

Cystic and necrotic metastases. Cystic and necrotic lymph node metastases in head and neck cancers are common, particularly with squamous cell carcinoma and papillary thyroid cancer. The cystic or necrotic components do not display ¹⁸FDG avidity (**Fig. 20**). There may be a rim of viable hypermetabolic tumor, which can nevertheless be inconspicuous on PET if sufficiently thin, hence the importance of referencing anatomic imaging.[34]

Lesion obscuration due to physiologic hypermetabolism. Malignant FDG-avid lesions adjacent to another ¹⁸FDG-avid lesion or normal structure with elevated metabolism may lead to a false-negative interpretation. This can be an issue for skull base tumors due to the high ¹⁸FDG activity of the brain (**Fig. 21**). Likewise, small tumors in the oropharynx can be obscured by the high physiologic activity of the tonsils and the high metabolic activity of extraocular muscles can obscure small lesions in the orbit. These pitfalls can be avoided through correlation with anatomic imaging, as well as the review of the fused PET/CT images in coronal and sagittal planes.

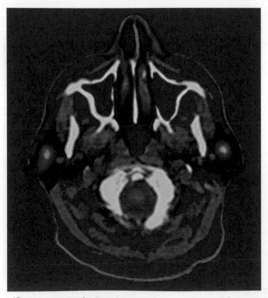

Fig. 18. Warthin tumors. Axial ¹⁸FDG-PET/CT fusion image shows bilateral hypermetabolic parotid tumors.

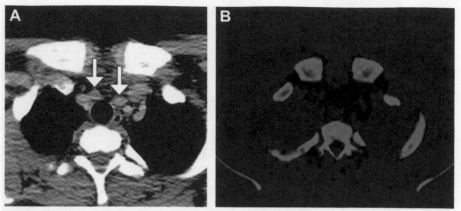

Fig. 19. Well-differentiated papillary thyroid cancer lymph node metastasis. Axial CT image (*A*) shows lymphadenopathy in the central compartment (*arrows*). There is no corresponding hypermetabolism of ^{18}FDG-PET (*B*).

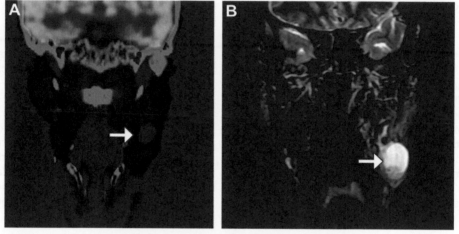

Fig. 20. Cystic lymph nodes. Coronal ^{18}FDG-PET/CT (*A*) and T2-weighted MRI (*B*) show large left suprahyoid lymph node with minimal peripheral hypermetabolism (*arrows*).

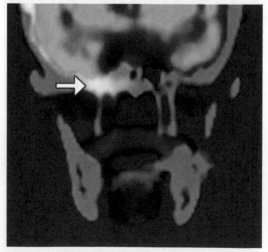

Fig. 21. Brain activity obscuring skull base tumor. Coronal ^{18}FDG-PET/CT image shows a hypermetabolic right skull base metastasis (*arrow*), obscured by adjacent high brain uptake.

CLINICS CARE POINTS

- Correlation with anatomic imaging is imperative for optimal interpreting head and neck 18FDG-PET.
- Potential false positive results include artifacts, normal physiologic activity, inflammatory/infectious conditions, treatment effects, and benign neoplasms.
- Potential negative positive results include inherently hypometabolic malignant neoplasms, cystic/necrotic metastases, and lesions obscured by normally high physiologic activity.

DISCLOSURE

The authors have nothing to disclose.

REFERENCES

1. Bernsdorf M, Loft A, Berthelsen AK, et al. FDG-PET/CT identified distant metastases and synchronous cancer in squamous cell carcinoma of the head and neck: the impact of smoking and P16-s. Eur Arch Otorhinolaryngol 2021. https://doi.org/10.1007/s00405-021-06890-7.
2. Stadler TM, Morand GB, Rupp NJ, et al. FDG-PET-CT/MRI in head and neck squamous cell carcinoma: Impact on pretherapeutic N classification, detection of distant metastases, and second primary tumors. Head Neck 2021;43(7):2058–68.
3. Boellaard R, O'Doherty MJ, Weber WA, et al. FDG PET and PET/CT: EANM procedure guidelines for tumour PET imaging: version 1.0. Eur J Nucl Med Mol Imaging 2010;37(1):181–200.
4. Kim Y, Roh JL, Kim JS, et al. Chest radiography or chest CT plus head and neck CT versus (18)F-FDG PET/CT for detection of distant metastasis and synchronous cancer in patients with head and neck cancer. Oral Oncol 2019;88:109–14.
5. Rangaswamy B, Fardanesh MR, Genden EM, et al. Improvement in the detection of locoregional recurrence in head and neck malignancies: F-18 fluorodeoxyglucose–positron emission tomography/computed tomography compared to high-resolution contrast-enhanced computed tomography and endoscopic examination. Laryngoscope 2013;123(11):2664–9. https://doi.org/10.1002/lary.24077.
6. Wong WL. PET-CT for Staging and Detection of Recurrence of Head and Neck Cancer. Semin Nucl Med 2021;51(1):13–25.
7. Goerres GW, Hany TF, Kamel E, et al. Head and neck imaging with PET and PET/CT: artefacts from dental metallic implants. Eur J Nucl Med Mol Imaging 2002;29(3):367–70.
8. Park JY, Lee YH. The Role of (18)F-FDG PET/CT for Evaluation of Cervical Metastatic Lymph Nodes in a Patient with Metallic Artifacts from Dental Prosthesis: a Case Report. Nucl Med Mol Imaging 2020;54(5):252–5.
9. Mihailovic J, Killeen RP, Duignan JA. PET/CT Variants and Pitfalls in Head and Neck Cancers Including Thyroid Cancer. Semin Nucl Med 2021;51(5):419–40.
10. Kim SY, Beer M, Tshering Vogel DW. Imaging in head and neck cancers: Update for non-radiologist. Oral Oncol 2021;120:105434.
11. Bhargava P, Rahman S, Wendt J. Atlas of confounding factors in head and neck PET/CT imaging. Clin Nucl Med 2011;36(5):e20–9.
12. Legot F, Tixier F, Hadzic M, et al. Use of baseline 18F-FDG PET scan to identify initial sub-volumes with local failure after concomitant radio-chemotherapy in head and neck cancer. Oncotarget 2018;9(31):21811–9.
13. Schöder H, Yeung HW, Gonen M, Kraus D, Larson SM. Head and neck cancer: clinical usefulness and accuracy of PET/CT image fusion. Radiology 2004;231(1):65–72.
14. Chaput A, Calais J, Robin P, et al. Correlation between fluorodeoxyglucose hotspots on pretreatment positron emission tomography/CT and preferential sites of local relapse after chemoradiotherapy for head and neck squamous cell carcinoma. Head Neck 2017;39(6):1155–65.
15. Kostakoglu L, Hardoff R, Mirtcheva R, Goldsmith SJ. PET-CT fusion imaging in differentiating physiologic from pathologic FDG uptake. Radiographics 2004;24(5):1411–31.
16. Blake MA, Singh A, Setty BN, et al. Pearls and pitfalls in interpretation of abdominal and pelvic PET-CT. Radiographics 2006;26(5):1335–53.
17. Beyer T, Tellmann L, Nickel I, Pietrzyk U. On the use of positioning aids to reduce misregistration in the head and neck in whole-body PET/CT studies. J Nucl Med 2005;46(4):596–602.
18. Ela Bella AJ, Zhang YR, Fan W, et al. Maximum standardized uptake value on PET/CT in preoperative assessment of lymph node metastasis from thoracic esophageal squamous cell carcinoma. Chin J Cancer 2014;33(4):211–7. https://doi.org/10.5732/cjc.013.10039.
19. Lyons K, Seghers V, Sorensen JI, et al. Comparison of Standardized Uptake Values in Normal Structures Between PET/CT and PET/MRI in a Tertiary Pediatric Hospital: A Prospective Study. AJR Am J Roentgenol 2015;205(5):1094–101.
20. Minamimoto R, Mosci C, Jamali M, Mittra E, Gambhir S, Iagaru A. Observed standardized uptake values in normal tissues and malignant lesions on combined 18F-NaF/18F-FDG PET/CT. Journal of Nuclear Medicine 2014;55(supplement 1):1638.

21. Nakamoto Y, Tatsumi M, Hammoud D, et al. Normal FDG Distribution Patterns in the Head and Neck: PET/CT Evaluation. Radiology 2005;234(3):879–85. https://doi.org/10.1148/radiol.2343030301.

22. Tsuchiya T, Osanai T, Ishikawa A, et al. Hibernomas show intense accumulation of FDG positron emission tomography. *J Comput Assist Tomogr* Mar-apr 2006;30(2):333–6. https://doi.org/10.1097/00004728-200603000-00033.

23. Rousseau C, Bourbouloux E, Campion L, et al. Brown fat in breast cancer patients: analysis of serial (18)F-FDG PET/CT scans. Eur J Nucl Med Mol Imaging 2006;33(7):785–91. https://doi.org/10.1007/s00259-006-0066-x.

24. Basu S, Houseni M, Alavi A. Significance of incidental fluorodeoxyglucose uptake in the parotid glands and its impact on patient management. Nucl Med Commun 2008;29(4):367–73. https://doi.org/10.1097/MNM.0b013e3282f8147a.

25. Ahmad Sarji S. Physiological uptake in FDG PET simulating disease. Biomed Imaging Interv J 2006; 2(4):e59. https://doi.org/10.2349/biij.2.4.e59.

26. Blodgett TM, Fukui MB, Snyderman CH, et al. Combined PET-CT in the head and neck: part 1. Physiologic, altered physiologic, and artifactual FDG uptake. Radiographics 2005;25(4):897–912. https://doi.org/10.1148/rg.254035156.

27. Roh JL, Ryu CH, Choi SH, et al. Clinical utility of 18F-FDG PET for patients with salivary gland malignancies. J Nucl Med 2007;48(2):240–6.

28. Cook GJ, Fogelman I, Maisey MN. Normal physiological and benign pathological variants of 18-fluoro-2-deoxyglucose positron-emission tomography scanning: potential for error in interpretation. Semin Nucl Med 1996;26(4):308–14. https://doi.org/10.1016/s0001-2998(96)80006-7.

29. Stahl A, Dzewas B, Schwaiger M, et al. Excretion of FDG into saliva and its significance for PET imaging. *Nuklearmedizin* Oct 2002;41(5):214–6.

30. Purohit BS, Ailianou A, Dulguerov N, et al. FDG-PET/CT pitfalls in oncological head and neck imaging. Insights Imaging 2014;5(5):585–602. https://doi.org/10.1007/s13244-014-0349-x.

31. Zhu Z, Chou C, Yen TC, et al. Elevated F-18 FDG uptake in laryngeal muscles mimicking thyroid cancer metastases. Clin Nucl Med 2001;26(8):689–91. https://doi.org/10.1097/00003072-200108000-00005.

32. Zhuang H, Yu JQ, Alavi A. Applications of fluorodeoxyglucose-PET imaging in the detection of infection and inflammation and other benign disorders. Radiol Clin North Am 2005;43(1):121–34. https://doi.org/10.1016/j.rcl.2004.07.005.

33. Meerwein CM, Queiroz M, Kollias S, et al. Post-treatment surveillance of head and neck cancer: pitfalls in the interpretation of FDG PET-CT/MRI. Swiss Med Wkly 2015;145:w14116. https://doi.org/10.4414/smw.2015.14116.

34. Lee N, Yoo Ie R, Park SY, et al. Significance of Incidental Nasopharyngeal Uptake on (18)F-FDG PET/CT: Patterns of Benign/Physiologic Uptake and Differentiation from Malignancy. Nucl Med Mol Imaging 2015;49(1):11–8. https://doi.org/10.1007/s13139-014-0299-8.

35. Fukui MB, Blodgett TM, Snyderman CH, et al. Combined PET-CT in the head and neck: part 2. Diagnostic uses and pitfalls of oncologic imaging. Radiographics 2005;25(4):913–30. https://doi.org/10.1148/rg.254045136.

36. Boss A, Stegger L, Bisdas S, et al. Feasibility of simultaneous PET/MR imaging in the head and upper neck area. Eur Radiol 2011;21(7):1439–46. https://doi.org/10.1007/s00330-011-2072-z.

37. Liu Y. Postoperative reactive lymphadenitis: A potential cause of false-positive FDG PET/CT. World J Radiol 2014;6(12):890–4. https://doi.org/10.4329/wjr.v6.i12.890.

38. Nakagawa T, Yamada M, Suzuki Y. 18F-FDG uptake in reactive neck lymph nodes of oral cancer: relationship to lymphoid follicles. J Nucl Med 2008;49(7):1053–9. https://doi.org/10.2967/jnumed.107.049718.

39. Kapoor V, Fukui MB, McCook BM. Role of 18FFDG PET/CT in the Treatment of Head and Neck Cancers: Posttherapy Evaluation and Pitfalls. Am J Roentgenol 2005;184(2):589–97. https://doi.org/10.2214/ajr.184.2.01840589.

40. Debnam JM, Garden AS, Ginsberg LE. Benign ulceration as a manifestation of soft tissue radiation necrosis: imaging findings. AJNR Am J Neuroradiol 2008; 29(3):558–62. https://doi.org/10.3174/ajnr.A0886.

41. Friedman ER, Saindane AM. Pitfalls in the staging of cancer of the major salivary gland neoplasms. Neuroimaging Clin N Am 2013;23(1):107–22. https://doi.org/10.1016/j.nic.2012.08.009.

42. Metser U, Miller E, Lerman H, et al. Benign nonphysiologic lesions with increased 18F-FDG uptake on PET/CT: characterization and incidence. AJR Am J Roentgenol 2007;189(5):1203–10. https://doi.org/10.2214/ajr.07.2083.

43. Horiuchi M, Yasuda S, Shohtsu A, et al. Four cases of Warthin's tumor of the parotid gland detected with FDG PET. Ann Nucl Med 1998;12(1):47–50. https://doi.org/10.1007/bf03165416.

44. Metser U, Even-Sapir E. Increased (18)F-fluorodeoxyglucose uptake in benign, nonphysiologic lesions found on whole-body positron emission tomography/computed tomography (PET/CT): accumulated data from four years of experience with PET/CT. Semin Nucl Med 2007;37(3):206–22. https://doi.org/10.1053/j.semnuclmed.2007.01.001.

45. Uchida Y, Minoshima S, Kawata T, et al. Diagnostic value of FDG PET and salivary gland scintigraphy for parotid tumors. Clin Nucl Med 2005;30(3):170–6. https://doi.org/10.1097/00003072-200503000-00005.

Postsurgical and Postradiation Findings in the Head and Neck Imaging

Charles Pierce, MD, MS[a], Daniel T. Ginat, MD, MS[b],*

KEYWORDS

• Surgery • Radiation • Imaging • Head • Neck

KEY POINTS

- Head and neck surgery can produce identifiable findings on imaging that can be distinguished from unrelated abnormalities by knowing the proper context and typical set of actions that lead to the changes observed.
- Radiation therapy in the head and neck can lead to various complications, often with a substantially delayed onset, that can confound the image interpretation.
- Consulting available clinical records and other imaging modalities can help clarify what is encountered on the posttreatment scans.

INTRODUCTION

There is a wide variety of surgical procedures and radiation therapy effects that may be observed on head and neck imaging. These interventions can lead to altered anatomy and complications that can confound the interpretation of the images. The purpose of this article is to review selected surgical procedures and radiation therapy effects and their potential mimics.

COSMETIC FACIAL FILLERS

Augmentation of the facial soft tissues for cosmetic purposes can be accomplished using a variety of injectable agents, such as calcium hydroxyapatite–based gels, which appear as dense bone attenuation (**Fig. 1**).[1] These fillers can resorb over time and become less conspicuous. Other facial fillers, such as collagen and hyaluronic acid gels, appear as nearly fluid attenuation. The MR imaging characteristics of facial fillers are variable, but those with a high water content display high T2 and low T1 signal (**Fig. 2**).[1] In addition, facial fillers can display associated enhancement and hypermetabolism on PET with fludeoxyglucose F 18 ([18]FDG-PET), particularly in the setting of infection and foreign body granuloma formation.[1] Thus, potential mimics of facial fillers and implants and their complications on imaging may include cellulitis, neoplasms, and hematomas (**Fig. 3**).

FACIAL REANIMATION

There are various static and dynamic reanimation procedures that can be performed for treating patients with facial nerve paralysis, including insertion of flaps, grafts, and slings.[2] For example, the gracilis muscle is often used as a graft and can appear as linear soft tissue strands that may extend from the zygoma to the oral commissure (**Fig. 4**).[2] The reconstructed tissues should not be mistaken for neoplasms (**Fig. 5**).

INTRAOCULAR SILICONE OIL

Retinal detachment can be treated by injection of intraocular silicone oil.[3,4] On computed tomography (CT), the silicone oil appears as globular and

[a] University of Illinois at Chicago, 1740 W Taylor Street, Chicago, IL 60612, USA; [b] Department of Radiology, University of Chicago, 5841 S Maryland Avenue, Chicago, IL 60637, USA
* Corresponding author.
E-mail address: dtg1@uchicago.edu

Neuroimag Clin N Am 32 (2022) 299–313
https://doi.org/10.1016/j.nic.2022.01.003

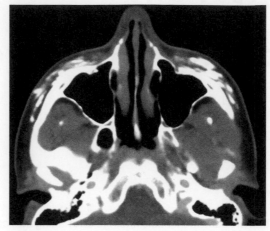

Fig. 1. Hydroxyapatite fillers. Axial CT image shows streaky hyperattenuating material within the bilateral cheek subcutaneous tissues, which correspond to the calcium hydroxyapatite filler.

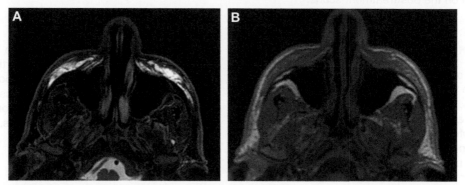

Fig. 2. Gel-based cosmetic fillers. Axial fat-suppressed T2-weighted (*A*) and T1-weighted (*B*) MR images show material with fluid signal in the bilateral cheek subcutaneous tissues.

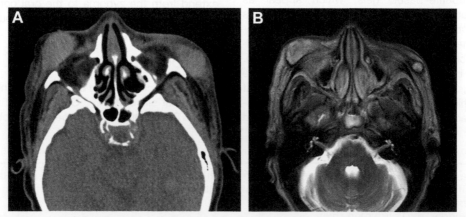

Fig. 3. Facial hematomas. Axial CT (*A*) and T2-weighted MR imaging (*B*) show hematomas in the bilateral cheeks from trauma.

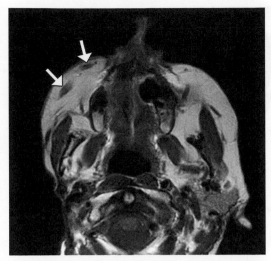

Fig. 4. Facial reanimation. The patient underwent right parotidectomy for tumor resection with facial nerve sacrifice. Axial T1-weighted MR imaging shows right facial subcutaneous tissue muscle grafts (*arrows*).

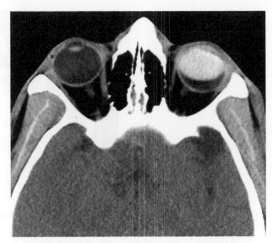

Fig. 6. Intraocular silicone oil. Axial CT image shows hyperattenuating material floating within the left globe. The lens is also absent.

hyperattenuating, measuring up to approximately 130 HU (**Fig. 6**), and should not be confused with tumor or hemorrhage (**Fig. 7**).[4] Paradoxically, the silicone oil floats, which is a characteristic distinguishing feature.[3,4] On MR imaging, chemical shift artifacts can be observed along the margins of the oil (see Marshall and colleagues' article, "Magnetic Resonance Imaging (MRI) Artifacts in the Head and Neck Region: Pitfalls and Solutions," in this issue).

PNEUMATIC RETINOPEXY

Retinal detachment can also be treated by injection of gas into the vitreous.[3] The bubble of gas is readily depicted on CT with an associated fluid level (**Fig. 8**)[3,5]; this should not be mistaken for pneumo-orbit from trauma (**Fig. 9**) or infection. Depending on the particular type of gas used, the bubble can last several days to weeks.[3,5]

NASOSEPTAL FLAP

Skull base defects can be sealed using nearby nasal septal flaps.[6] These flaps have a characteristic imaging appearance, in which a thin sheet of enhancing tissue is folded backwards toward the

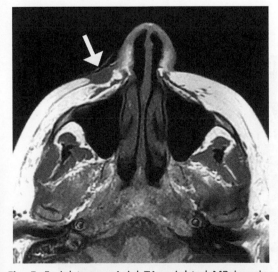

Fig. 5. Facial tumor. Axial T1-weighted MR imaging shows a mass in the right cheek (*arrow*), which represents a cutaneous carcinoma.

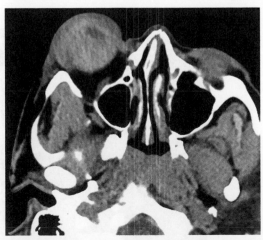

Fig. 7. Intraocular hemorrhage. Axial CT image shows extensive hyperattenuation within the right globe and associated preseptal swelling from trauma.

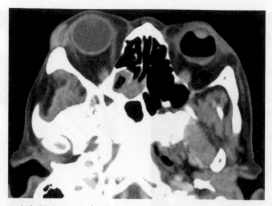

Fig. 8. Pneumatic retinopexy. Axial CT image shows gas within the posterior right globe.

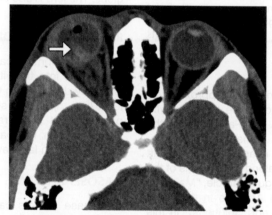

Fig. 9. Ruptured globe. Axial CT image shows a small amount of air in the right globe and a dislocated, hypoattenuating lens (*arrow*) secondary to BB pellet injury.

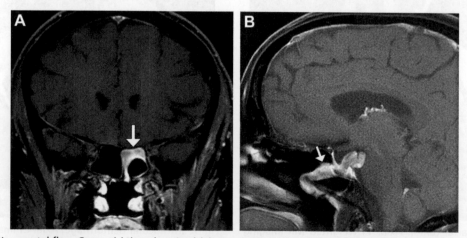

Fig. 10. Nasoseptal flap. Coronal (*A*) and sagittal (*B*) postcontrast T1-weighted MR images show enhancing tissue extending from the nasal septum to the floor of the sella (*arrows*).

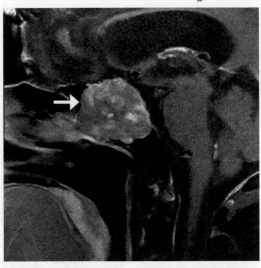

Fig. 11. Invasive pituitary tumor. Sagittal postcontrast T1-weighted MR imaging shows a pituitary mass that extends into the sphenoid sinuses (*arrow*).

skull base (Fig. 10).[6] These findings are generally distinguishable from neoplasm, which tends to be more nodular and typically does not enhance as avidly as the mucosa in the flap (Fig. 11).

CALDWELL-LUC PROCEDURE

In the past, the Caldwell-Luc procedure was performed to treat chronic sinusitis.[7,8] The procedure involved creating an opening in the lower nasoantral wall via an anterior maxillary sinus approach (Fig. 12).[7,8] The procedure is often complicated by fibro-osseous proliferation, which can mimic recurrent sinus disease, as well as sinus contraction, which can resemble maxillary sinus hypoplasia (Fig. 13).[8] Currently, variations of the Caldwell-Luc procedure may be implemented as an approach for sinonasal tumor resection.[9]

FRONTAL SINUS OBLITERATION

The frontal sinus can be obliterated for treating mucoceles, cerebrospinal fluid leakage, and tumors.[10] The frontal sinus can be sealed off from the rest of the paranasal sinuses using materials such as bone cement in the frontoethmoidal recess.[11] The cement used as part of the surgery is very hyperattenuating on CT (Fig. 14) and can resemble an osteoma on imaging (Fig. 15).

SINUS LIFT

The loss of teeth leads to resorption of alveolar bone. In order to perform dental reconstruction with osteointegrated implants, the alveolar bone may have to be built-up via the sinus lift procedure[12]; this can be achieved by depositing bone

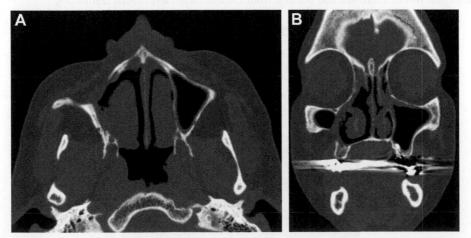

Fig. 12. Caldwell-Luc procedure. Axial (*A*) and coronal (*B*) CT images show defects in the anterior and medial right maxillary sinus walls. The right maxillary sinus is also contracted.

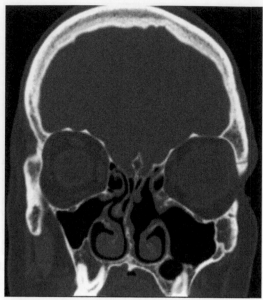

Fig. 13. Hypoplastic maxillary sinus. Coronal CT image shows a relatively small right maxillary sinus. There are also findings related to endoscopic sinus surgery on the left side.

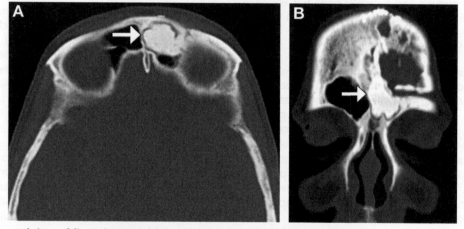

Fig. 14. Frontal sinus obliteration. Axial (*A*) and coronal (*B*) CT images show globular cement (*arrows*) in the left frontoethmoidal recess. There are also findings from the associated left frontal craniotomy.

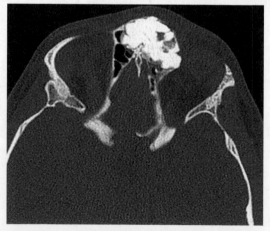

Fig. 15. Osteoma. Axial CT image shows a markedly hyperattenuating lobulated mass in the frontoethmoidal recesses.

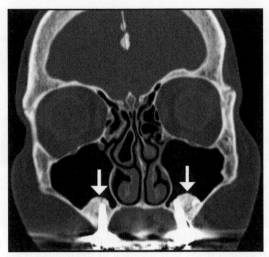

Fig. 16. Coronal CT image shows mounds of bone graft (*arrows*) along the alveolar recesses of the bilateral maxillary sinuses with embedded osteointegrated dental implants.

graft along the floor of the maxillary sinus, which appears as calcified mounds, often anchoring metal dental implants (**Fig. 16**).[12] The bone graft should not be mistaken for tumors or hyperostosis related to chronic sinusitis (**Fig. 17**).

INCUS INTERPOSITION

The incus can be used to reconstruct a partly eroded ossicular chain.[13] The procedure usually involves creating a notch in the short process of the incus and repositioning it between the malleus and remaining stapes superstructure, stapes prosthesis, or stapes footplate, along with additional remodeling of the long process depending on the

particular situation (**Fig. 18**).[13] The altered configuration of the ossicular chain should not be confused with traumatic dislocation on imaging, whereby the morphology of the incus would not be as drastically altered, even if also fractured (**Fig. 19**).

Tympanoplasty

Reconstruction of the tympanic membrane can be performed using cartilage grafts.[14] The cartilage graft appears as soft tissue attenuation on CT (**Fig. 20**); this usually has a sheetlike configuration but can sometimes appear more nodular and protrude into the middle ear cavity, which can

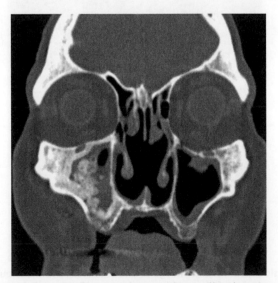

Fig. 17. Chronic sinusitis. Coronal CT image shows extensive right maxillary hyperostosis and mucosal thickening.

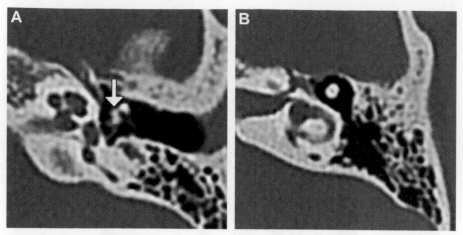

Fig. 18. Incus interposition. Axial CT images (*A, B*) show the sculpted incus (*arrow*) positioned in the mesotympanum rather than in the epitympanum, where only the head of the malleus resides.

potentially resemble recurrent cholesteatoma (**Fig. 21**).[14] Although this can usually be distinguished via otoscopy, MR imaging with diffusion-weighted imaging can help rule out cholesteatoma.[15]

VOCAL CORD AUGMENTATION

Vocal cord palsy can be treated via surgical medialization procedures with implants and injectable agents.[16,17] For example, injection laryngoplasty medializes the paralyzed vocal cord to improve glottis closure and competence.[16] Fat, collagen, hydroxyapatite, polytetrafluoroethylene, and absorbable gelatin powder are various substances that are injected for this purpose.[16] These substances are often identifiable on diagnostic

imaging and should not be misinterpreted as laryngeal masses or traumatically introduced foreign bodies. In particular, certain materials such as hydroxyapatite can stimulate local fibroblast activity and macrophage accumulation, leading to increased [18]FDG uptake on PET (**Fig. 22**), which can mimic activity associated with neoplasm (**Fig. 23**).[18]

GASTRIC PULL-UP

Esophageal cancer can be treated via esophagectomy, which in turn can be reconstructed via gastric pull-up.[19] There are many variations of the gastric pull-up surgical technique, but the operation essentially consists of repositioning the stomach in the chest and/or neck.[19] The displaced

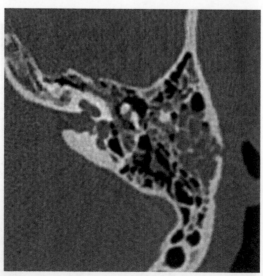

Fig. 19. Incudomalleolar dislocation. Axial CT image shows a detached left malleus head in the epitympanum. There is also a fracture through the left mastoid bone with opacification of the air cells.

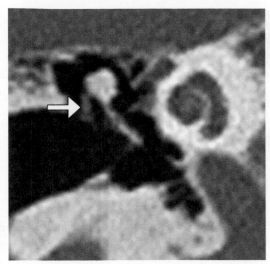

Fig. 20. Tympanoplasty. Coronal CT image shows an area of soft tissue thickening along the upper portion of the reconstructed tympanic membrane, which corresponds to the cartilage graft (*arrow*).

stomach can be recognized on imaging by the presence of characteristic rugae within the lumen (**Fig. 24**). On occasion, the gastric pull-up can appear masslike or partially collapsed with areas of trapped air or fluid, which can mimic neoplasm or abscess (**Fig. 25**). If there is any ambiguity, endoscopy can be useful.

MYOCUTANEOUS FLAPS

Myocutaneous flaps can demonstrate persistent enhancement that can often be differentiated from tumor recurrence by the presence of muscle

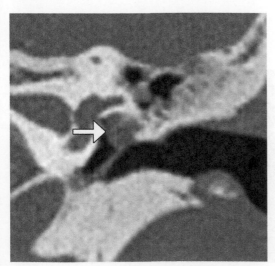

Fig. 21. Cholesteatoma. Coronal CT image shows an opacity in the left Prussak space (*arrow*).

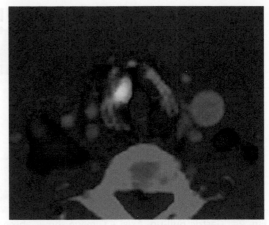

Fig. 22. Hydroxyapatite laryngeal augmentation. Axial fused [18]FDG-PET/CT image shows hypermetabolism associated with right vocal cord filler.

striations.[20] Pedicle flaps comprise a vascular supply consisting of an artery and at least one vein. On postcontrast CT, the vessels should enhance as other vascular structures (**Fig. 26**) and should not be misinterpreted as unintended or intended foreign bodies, such as iodoform gauze pads that are used for wound debridement (**Fig. 27**). If there is any uncertainty regarding the nature of the vascular pedicle and whether it is patent, Doppler ultrasound may be performed.

POSTSURGICAL DENERVATION

Various nerves can be injured during head and neck dissection, leading to denervation changes in the muscles supplied by the nerves. The initial signs of denervation include high T2 signal and

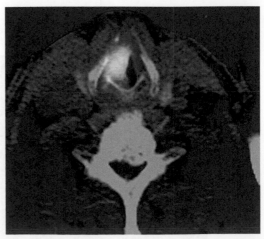

Fig. 23. Laryngeal squamous cell carcinoma. Axial fused [18]FDG-PET/CT image shows hypermetabolism associated with a right vocal cord tumor.

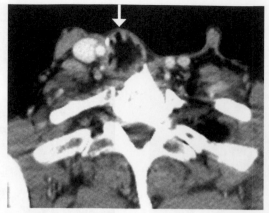

Fig. 24. Gastric pull-up. Axial CT image shows absence of the cervical esophagus and reconstruction using the stomach in the anterior neck (*arrow*). The rugae are visible within the lumen of the transposed stomach.

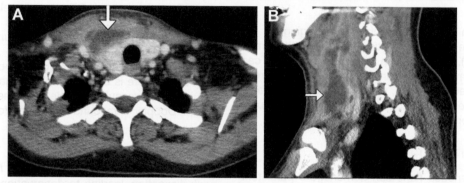

Fig. 25. Neck abscess. Axial (*A*) and sagittal (*B*) CT images show an elongated, irregular, rim-enhancing fluid collection in the right anterior visceral space (*arrows*).

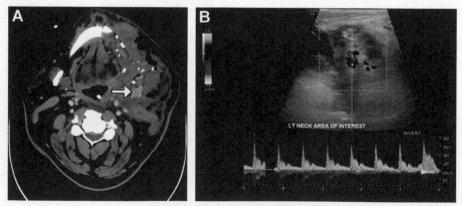

Fig. 26. Vascular pedicle. Axial CT image (*A*) shows a 3-vessel pedicle, consisting of the peroneal artery together with 2 vena comitans (*arrow*). Doppler ultrasound (*B*) shows corresponding arterial flow in the peroneal artery.

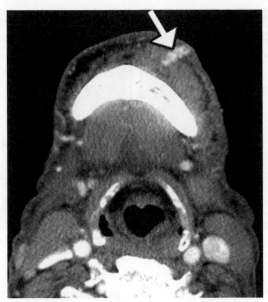

Fig. 27. Iodoform gauze. Axial CT image shows hyperattenuating material in a left lower face open wound (*arrow*).

enhancement of the affected tissues (**Fig. 28**), which can potentially resemble neoplasm (**Fig. 29**).[21] However, the denervated tissues respect the anatomic boundaries and lack significant mass effect.[21] Ultimately, denervation injury leads to muscle atrophy with fatty infiltration.[21]

RADIATION-INDUCED NECROSIS

Radiation therapy can lead to necrosis of head and neck tissues, particularly the brain and laryngeal cartilages. Chondroradionecrosis can manifest as lysis and fragmentation of the cartilage, which can be accompanied by regional soft tissue swelling and pockets of gas (**Fig. 30**).[22] Brain necrosis can appear as a peripherally enhancing lesion with surrounding vasogenic edema, usually in the anterior temporal lobe in cases of head and neck cancer treated with radiation (**Fig. 31**).[23] Although glioblastomas and brain metastases can occur in patients with head and neck cancer and can potentially resemble radiation necrosis on MR imaging, these tend to display hypermetabolism on PET.[24,25] Alternatively, abscess can resemble the ring enhancement and vasogenic edema associated with radiation necrosis (**Fig. 32**).

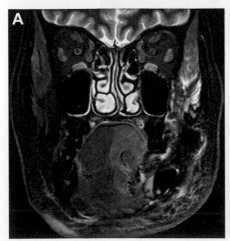
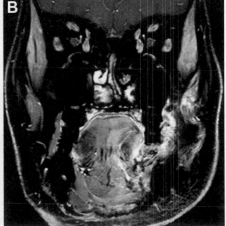

Fig. 28. Hypoglossal denervation. Coronal fat-suppressed T2-weighted (*A*) and postcontrast T1-weighted (*B*) MR images show edema and enhancement in the left hemitongue.

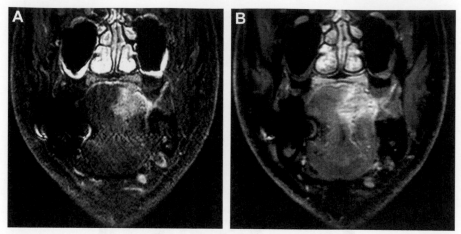

Fig. 29. Tongue cancer. Coronal fat-suppressed T2-weighted (*A*) and postcontrast T1-weighted (*B*) MR images show an infiltrative and enhancing left tongue mass.

CAROTID BLOWOUT SYNDROME

Carotid blowout syndrome is a potential complication of radiation therapy in which there is rupture of the vessel, and this can manifest as exposed artery, associated necrotic or viable tumor, pseudoaneurysm, or frank contrast extravasation on CT angiography (**Fig. 33**).[26] Catheter angiography can be useful for confirming and managing carotid blowout.[26] However, intermittent bleeding can be a pitfall of impending carotid blowout

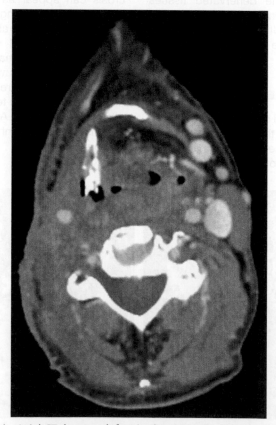

Fig. 30. Chondroradionecrosis. Axial CT shows a defect in the posterior right thyroid cartilage with surrounding pockets of gas and regional soft tissue swelling.

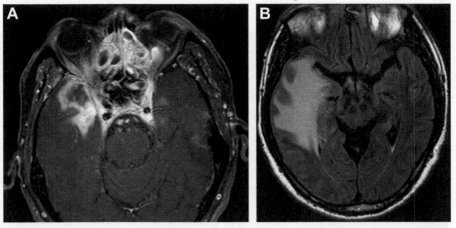

Fig. 31. Radiation-induced brain necrosis. Axial postcontrast T1-weighted (*A*) and axial T2-weighted FLAIR (*B*) MR images show a central area of necrosis within a peripherally enhancing area and surrounding vasogenic edema in the right temporal lobe.

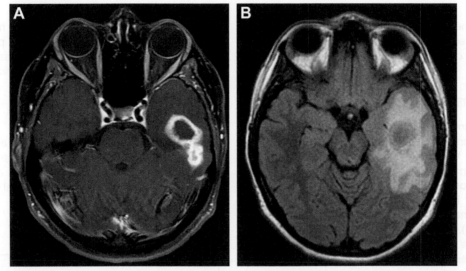

Fig. 32. Brain abscess. Axial postcontrast T1-weighted (*A*) and T2-weighted FLAIR (*B*) MR images show a ring-enhancing lesion in the left temporal lobe with surrounding vasogenic edema.

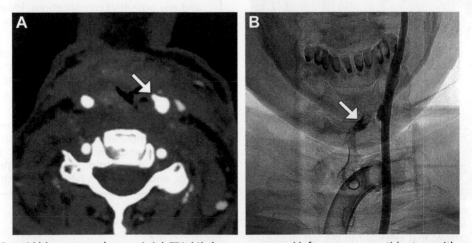

Fig. 33. Carotid blowout syndrome. Axial CTA (*A*) shows an exposed left common carotid artery with a pseudoaneurysm (*arrow*) in a patient with head and neck cancer status postradiation and surgery. Conventional angiography (*B*) shows a small pseudoaneurysm along the left common carotid artery with extravasation of contrast (*arrow*).

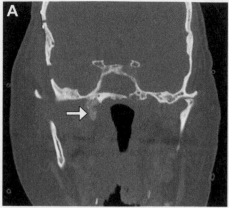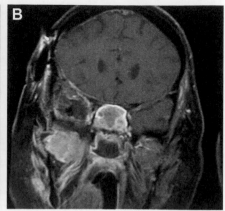

Fig. 34. Radiation-induced sarcoma. Coronal CT (*A*) shows abnormal bone formation in the right infratemporal fossa (*arrow*). Coronal fat-suppressed postcontrast T1-weighted MR imaging (*B*) shows an associated enhancing mass (high-grade sarcomatous tumor with osteosarcomatous and rhabdomyosarcomatous differentiation).

syndrome, which is why the condition of the soft tissues surrounding the artery in cross-sectional imaging can serve as an important indicator.

RADIOTHERAPY-RELATED SECONDARY TUMORS

Neoplasms can occasionally be caused by radiation therapy, usually with a latency of many years.[27] Various histologies of radiation-induced neoplasms can be encountered in the head and neck, most commonly fibrosarcoma and osteosarcoma.[28] The presence of hyperostosis in an otherwise enhancing mass can suggest osteosarcoma (**Fig. 34**).[29] Otherwise, the differential diagnosis depends on location, with radiation-induced tumors being more remote from the site of the

original neoplasm, particularly at the margin of the radiation field.[29,30] Otherwise, perineural spread should be considered as a possibility for a tumor located remote to the original primary cancer (**Fig. 35**).

SUMMARY

The results of various types of surgery and radiation therapy can have confounding imaging findings. Familiarity with these treatment effects in the head and neck can facilitate optimal radiological interpretation.

CLINICS CARE POINTS

- The goal of post-treatment imaging is to appropriately recognize what was performed and any potential complications, ideally with the assistance of relevant clinical information if needed.

- Head and neck surgery can alter the anatomy and physiology in such a way that these can mimic lesions, but often have distinctive imaging features and patient history that can help identify these appropriately.

- Radiation therapy in the head and neck can lead to complications that can mimic tumor recurrence and other abnormalities, but the particular distribution, subtle imaging features, and timing can help distinguish.

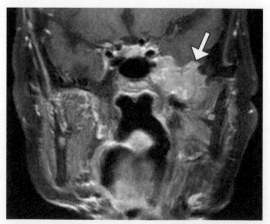

Fig. 35. Perineural tumor spread. Coronal postcontrast fat-suppressed T1-weighted MR imaging shows a tumor (*arrow*) that extends into the left middle cranial fossa in a patient with a history of adenoid cystic carcinoma.

DISCLOSURE

The authors have nothing to disclose.

REFERENCES

1. Ginat DT, Schatz CJ. Imaging features of midface injectable fillers and associated complications. AJNR Am J Neuroradiol 2013;34(8):1488–95.

2. Ginat DT, Bhama P, Cunnane ME, et al. Facial reanimation procedures depicted on radiologic imaging. AJNR Am J Neuroradiol 2014;35(9):1662–6.

3. Adams A, Mankad K, Poitelea C, et al. Post-operative orbital imaging: a focus on implants and prosthetic devices. Neuroradiology 2014;56(11):925–35.

4. Mathews VP, Elster AD, Barker PB, et al. Intraocular silicone oil: in vitro and in vivo MR and CT characteristics. AJNR Am J Neuroradiol 1994;15(2):343–7.

5. Lane JI, Watson RE, Witte RJ, et al. Retinal detachment: imaging of surgical treatments and complications. Radiographics 2003;23(4):983–94.

6. Kang MD, Escott E, Thomas AJ, et al. The MR imaging appearance of the vascular pedicle nasoseptal flap. AJNR Am J Neuroradiol 2009;30(4):781–6.

7. Unger JM, Dennison BF, Duncavage JA, et al. The radiological appearance of the post-Caldwell-Luc maxillary sinus. Clin Radiol 1986;37(1):77–81.

8. Nemec SF, Peloschek P, Koelblinger C, et al. Sinonasal imaging after Caldwell-Luc surgery: MDCT findings of an abandoned procedure in times of functional endoscopic sinus surgery. Eur J Radiol 2009;70(1):31–4.

9. Alim BM, Jomah M, Al-Thobaiti M. Maxillary sinus schwannoma. BMJ Case Rep 2018;2018.

10. Murphy J, Jones NS. Frontal sinus obliteration. J Laryngol Otol 2004;118(8):637–9.

11. Petruzzelli GJ, Stankiewicz JA. Frontal sinus obliteration with hydroxyapatite cement. Laryngoscope 2002;112(1):32–6.

12. Abrahams JJ, Hayt MW, Rock R. Sinus lift procedure of the maxilla in patients with inadequate bone for dental implants: radiographic appearance. AJR Am J Roentgenol 2000;174(5):1289–92.

13. Stone JA, Mukherji SK, Jewett BS, et al. CT evaluation of prosthetic ossicular reconstruction procedures: what the otologist needs to know. Radiographics 2000;20(3):593–605.

14. Williams MT, Ayache D. Imaging of the postoperative middle ear. Eur Radiol 2004;14(3):482–95.

15. Lingam RK, Bassett P. A meta-analysis on the diagnostic performance of non-echoplanar diffusion-weighted imaging in detecting middle ear cholesteatoma: 10 Years On. Otol Neurotol 2017;38(4):521–8.

16. Vachha BA, Ginat DT, Mallur P, et al. "Finding a voice": imaging features after phonosurgical procedures for vocal fold paralysis. AJNR Am J Neuroradiol 2016;37(9):1574–80.

17. Kumar VA, Lewin JS, Ginsberg LE. CT assessment of vocal cord medialization. AJNR Am J Neuroradiol 2006;27(8):1643–6.

18. Halpern BS, Britz-Cunningham SH, Kim CK. Intense focal F-18 FDG uptake in vocal cord associated with injection of calcium hydroxylapatite microspheres. Clin Nucl Med 2011;36(11):e175–7.

19. Flanagan JC, Batz R, Saboo SS, et al. Esophagectomy and Gastric Pull-through Procedures: Surgical Techniques, Imaging Features, and Potential Complications. Radiographics 2016;36(1):107–21.

20. Sedrak P, Lee PS, Guha-Thakurta N, et al. MRI findings of myocutaneous and fasciocutaneous flaps used for reconstruction of orbital exenteration defects. Ophthal Plast Reconstr Surg 2014;30(4):328–36.

21. Borges A. Imaging of denervation in the head and neck. Eur J Radiol 2010;74(2):378–90.

22. Roh J-L. Chondroradionecrosis of the larynx: diagnostic and therapeutic measures for saving the organ from radiotherapy sequelae. Clin Exp Otorhinolaryngol 2009;2(3):115–9.

23. Ali FS, Arevalo O, Zorofchian S, et al. Cerebral Radiation Necrosis: Incidence, Pathogenesis, Diagnostic Challenges, and Future Opportunities. Curr Oncol Rep 2019;21(8):66.

24. Horky LL, Hsiao EM, Weiss SE, et al. Dual phase FDG-PET imaging of brain metastases provides superior assessment of recurrence versus posttreatment necrosis. J Neurooncol 2011;103(1):137–46.

25. van Dijken BRJ, van Laar PJ, Smits M, et al. Perfusion MRI in treatment evaluation of glioblastomas: Clinical relevance of current and future techniques. J Magn Reson Imaging 2019;49(1):11–22.

26. Lee C-W, Yang C-Y, Chen Y-F, et al. CT angiography findings in carotid blowout syndrome and its role as a predictor of 1-year survival. AJNR Am J Neuroradiol 2014;35(3):562–7.

27. Braunstein S, Nakamura JL. Radiotherapy-induced malignancies: review of clinical features, pathobiology, and evolving approaches for mitigating risk. Front Oncol 2013;3:73.

28. Yamanaka R, Hayano A. Radiation-Induced Sarcomas of the Central Nervous System: A Systematic Review. World Neurosurg 2017;98:818–28.e7.

29. Cai P, Wu Y, Li L, et al. CT and MRI of radiation-induced sarcomas of the head and neck following radiotherapy for nasopharyngeal carcinoma. Clin Radiol 2013;68(7):683–9.

30. Abrigo JM, King AD, Leung SF, et al. MRI of radiation-induced tumors of the head and neck in post-radiation nasopharyngeal carcinoma. Eur Radiol 2009;19(5):1197–205.

Implants and Foreign Bodies on Head and Neck Imaging

Daniel T. Ginat, MD, MS

KEYWORDS

• Head • Neck • Foreign bodies • Implants • Imaging

KEY POINTS

- Although foreign bodies often have characteristic radiological features, some of these can be inconspicuous or mimic other things such as tumors.
- Familiarity with the uses and normal imaging appearances of surgical implants found in the head and neck can help to avoid misinterpreting what these are.
- Silicone is a commonly used material for implants in the head and neck and appears hyperattenuating on CT.
- Most metal surgical implants can safely undergo MRI, although some of these produce noticeable artifacts that degrade image quality.

INTRODUCTION

There are a wide variety of surgical implants and foreign bodies that may be observed on head and neck imaging. Although these materials generally have characteristic features, the lack of awareness of these items can confound the interpretation of the images. The purpose of this article is to review selected surgical implants and foreign body effects and their potential mimics, as well as address concerns regarding MR imaging compatibility.

COMESTIBLE FOREIGN BODY

Patients sometimes leave intraoral comestible foreign bodies in the oral cavity during a head and neck scan. Hard comestible foreign bodies tend to be hyperattenuating, potentially resembling tumors or calculi, whereas soft comestible foreign bodies tend to be heterogeneous and can be mistaken for mucosal lesions or abscess when foci of gas are present within chewable foreign bodies (**Fig. 1**).[1,2] To avoid misdiagnosis, patients should be asked to remove any intraoral foreign bodies before imaging.

WOOD

On computed tomography (CT), wood has been described as low attenuating or high attenuating, depending on the degree of air or other substances trapped within its cellulose matrix (**Fig. 2**).[3] On MR imaging, wood has the same signal intensity as air on all sequences. However, the linear configuration of wood can help differentiate this from air. Furthermore, the use of wide bone window settings on CT can also help in differentiating the two.

GLASS

CT can readily demonstrate even small glass fragments that might be embedded in the soft tissues, with attenuation in the range of 500 to 1900 HU (**Fig. 3**),[4] thereby potentially resembling bone fragments or gravel. On MR imaging, glass tends to display low T1 and T2 signals, along with susceptibility effect.

PLASTIC

Most plastic polymers display low attenuation on CT (**Fig. 4**).[5] Plastic appears echogenic on

Department of Radiology, University of Chicago, 5841 S Maryland Avenue, Chicago, IL 60637, USA
E-mail address: dtg1@uchicago.edu

Neuroimag Clin N Am 32 (2022) 315–326
https://doi.org/10.1016/j.nic.2022.01.004
1052-5149/22/

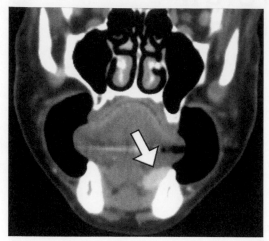

Fig. 1. Coronal computed tomographic (CT) image shows hyperattenuating material along the left floor of mouth (*arrow*), which corresponds to chewing gum.

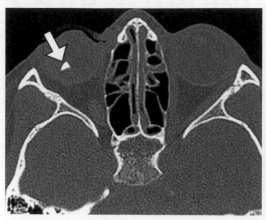

Fig. 3. Axial CT image shows a hyperattenuating glass fragment (*arrow*) in the right globe introduced by trauma.

ultrasonography but can be inconspicuous on MR imaging due to low signal on all sequences.

METAL

Although metals are highly hyperattenuating on CT, some are more so than others. For example, titanium tends not to produce significant streak and susceptibility artifact, whereas many other metals, such as those used in dental amalgam, create a lot of artifact on imaging (Fig. 5). In addition, titanium tends to produce fewer artifacts than other metals, such as steel, on MR imaging.[6]

COSMETIC IMPLANTS

Implants used for cosmetic facial surgery are often composed of silicon, particularly for chin and

cheek augmentation and rhinoplasty. The implants appear as high attenuation on CT and are generally shaped to fit the contours of the underlying maxillofacial skeleton or the soft tissues of the nose (Fig. 6). Although they might be encountered incidentally, imaging can be specifically performed to assess for associated complications, such as migration, infection, extrusion, foreign body reaction, heterotopic bone formation, and bone erosion.[7,8]

EYELID WEIGHTS

Facial nerve palsy can affect eye closure and lead to desiccation of the cornea. To prevent this

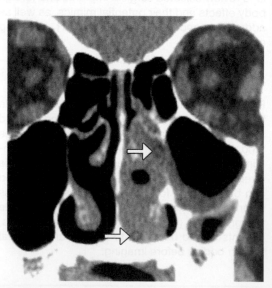

Fig. 4. Coronal CT image shows portions of a hypoattenuating bent plastic pen cartridge in cross section (*arrows*) with the hyperattenuating ink centrally lodged in the left nasal cavity.

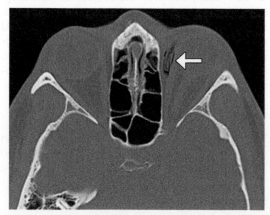

Fig. 2. Axial CT image shows a linear low-attenuation wood fragment (*arrow*) in the left orbit.

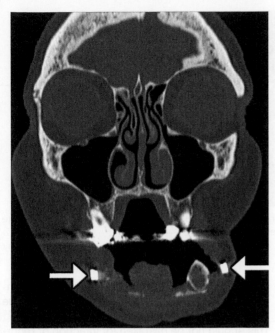

Fig. 5. Coronal CT image shows titanium mandibular plates (*arrows*) without streak artifact, unlike the maxillary dental amalgam.

complication, weights can be implanted into the upper eyelid. Eyelid weights are often composed of gold or platinum and produce considerable beam hardening artifacts on CT (**Fig. 7**), but are considered MR imaging safe.[9] Otherwise, the weights have a characteristic slightly curved rectangular shape, typically with small perforations that can help distinguish them from other foreign bodies.[10]

Eyelid Springs

Springs are also used for treating eyelid closure problems in the setting of facial nerve palsy.[10] These appear as metal wires with one limb along the superolateral orbital rim and another within the superior eyelid (**Fig. 8**). Radiographs are adequate for evaluating the integrity of the device.

SCLERAL BUCKLES

Scleral buckles can be used for treating retinal detachment. Hydrogel scleral buckles are no longer used, but may still be encountered in patients who undergo diagnostic imaging. These implants tend to swell with fluid and cause mass effect upon the orbital contents and can migrate.[11] The implants display fluid signal on MR imaging and when fragmented can mimic lesions, such as dermoid cysts (**Fig. 9**). However, the hydrogel fragments tend to have more rectilinear margins that can help differentiate them from natural lesions. At present, silicone scleral buckles are used, which can partially or completely encircle the globe in the coronal plane.[12] Silicone sponge scleral buckles display air attenuation on CT, whereas silicone rubber scleral buckles have high attenuation on CT (**Fig. 10**). The buckles normally indent the globe.

GLAUCOMA DRAINAGE DEVICES

A variety of implants can be used to treat complicated and refractory cases of glaucoma. Glaucoma tube shunts and valves consist of a plate positioned along the surface of the globe and a tube that enters that anterior chamber. There are several types of these glaucoma drainage devices, such as the Ahmed valve and the Baerveldt shunt. The devices are composed of a plastic that appears as low attenuation, unless they are impregnated with radioattenuating barium (**Fig. 11**). These devices are often associated with a fluid bleb, which can mimic orbital cystic lesions.[13] Alternatively, the EX-PRESS (Alcon Laboratories, Fort Worth, TX, USA) Mini glaucoma shunt is a stainless steel implant nearly 3 mm long and can shunt aqueous from the anterior chamber to a subconjunctival compartment in the anterior globe (**Fig. 12**).[14] These metallic devices should not be

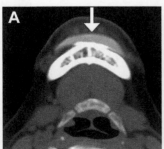
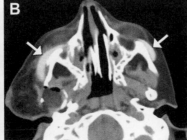
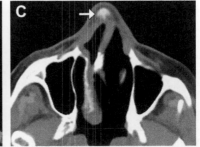

Fig. 6. Axial CT image (*A*) shows a chin implant (*arrow*). Axial CT image (*B*) shows bilateral cheek implants (*arrows*). Axial CT image (*C*) shows a rhinoplasty implant (*arrow*).

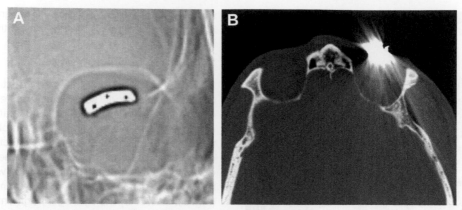

Fig. 7. Scout image (*A*) shows a slightly curved rectangular eyelid weight with small perforations. Axial CT image (*B*) shows extensive streak artifact associated with the eyelid weight.

mistaken for unintended foreign bodies or otherwise innocuous scleral calcifications.

OCULAR IMPLANTS

Ocular implants can be composed of solid or porous materials, such as coral-derived hydroxyapatite and porous polyethylene (Medpor, Porex Surgical, Inc, College Park, GA). Porous materials enable fibrovascular growth from the surrounding tissues into the porous implant, which ensures integration into the surrounding orbital tissues and reduces the incidence of complications such as exposure, extrusion, and infection. Postcontrast MR imaging can depict fibrovascular tissue ingrowth within the porous implants (**Fig. 13**).[15] This should not be mistaken for infection or recurrent tumor, which would be expected to appear as enhancement beyond the implant.

DACRYOCYSTOSTOMY TUBES

Epiphora caused by nasolacrimal duct stenosis can be treated by insertion of nasolacrimal duct tubes.[16] CT is sometimes performed to evaluate for proper positioning of the tube, which is from the inferomedial orbit to the inferior nasal cavity. The tubes appear as hyperattenuating structures with a flange on the upper end on CT (**Fig. 14**). Sometimes these tubes can become dislodged.

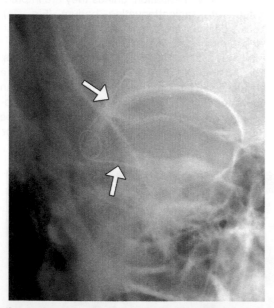

Fig. 8. Frontal radiograph shows the 2 limbs of the fine metallic wire spring (*arrows*) projecting over the right superolateral orbit.

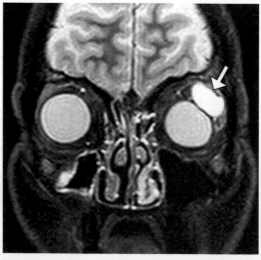

Fig. 9. Coronal T2-weighted MR imaging shows the expanded hydrated hydrogel scleral buckle (*arrow*).

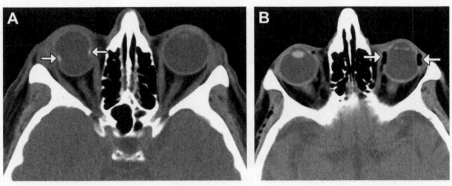

Fig. 10. Coronal CT image (*A*) shows a hyperattenuating silicone rubber scleral buckle encircling the right globe (*arrows*). Coronal CT image (*B*) shows a hypoattenuating silicone sponge scleral buckle encircling the left globe (*arrows*).

NASAL SEPTAL PROSTHESIS

Perforations of the nasal septum can cause sensations of nasal congestion and whistling sounds. The defects can be repaired using nasal septal button prostheses composed of materials such as silastic.[17] These implants appear as parallel hyperattenuating plates connected together in the middle (**Fig. 15**).

OSSICULAR PROSTHESES

A variety of alloplastic implants are available for reconstruction of the ossicular chain; these are often categorized as stapes prosthesis, partial ossicular replacement prosthesis, or total ossicular replacement prosthesis.[18] The appearance

on CT depends on the materials used, such as hydroxyapatite, metal, or plastic polymers (**Fig. 16**). Prosthesis complications that can be observed on CT include displacement, intravestibular protrusion, breakage, and postoperative granuloma or fibrosis formation. Some of the thin prostheses can resemble monopod stapes.

COCHLEAR IMPLANTS

There are a variety of cochlear implant models that are commercially available and consist of electrode arrays with multiple contacts that are inserted into the cochlea. Although the electrode and contacts are typically fully visible on CT, one particular model, the HiFocus Mid-Scala (Advanced Bionics, Valencia, CA), includes 16

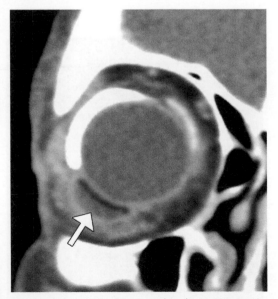

Fig. 11. Coronal CT shows a thin hyperattenuating superonasal Ahmed valve, a thick hyperattenuating superotemporal Baerveldt shunt, and an inferotemporal low-attenuation Ahmed valve with an associated fluid bleb (*arrow*).

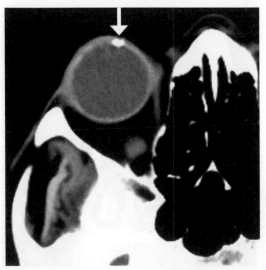

Fig. 12. Axial CT image shows the punctate metallic EX-PRESS glaucoma shunt in the anterior globe (*arrow*).

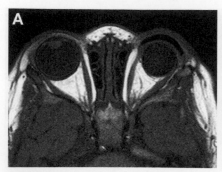

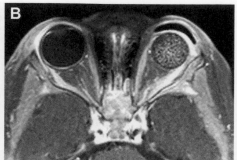

Fig. 13. Axial T1-weighted (*A*) and postcontrast T1-weighted (*B*) MR images show enhancement within the left orbital Medpor implant with relative sparing of the central portion.

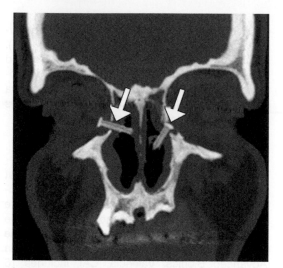

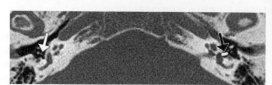

Fig. 16. Axial temporal bone CT image show a plastic stapes wire prosthesis on the right (*white arrow*) and a metallic stapes prosthesis on the left (*black arrow*).

Fig. 14. Coronal CT image shows the hyperattenuating nasolacrimal duct tubes (*arrows*).

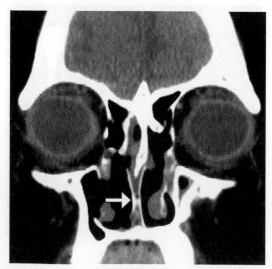

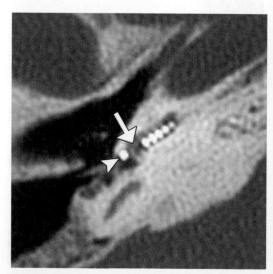

Fig. 17. Axial CT image shows an Advanced Bionics cochlear implant with a lucent gap (*arrow*) between the functioning electrode array contacts within the cochlea and the dummy contact within the round window niche (*arrowhead*).

Fig. 15. Coronal CT image shows the hyperattenuating plates of the nasal septal prosthesis (*arrow*) along a nasal septal defect.

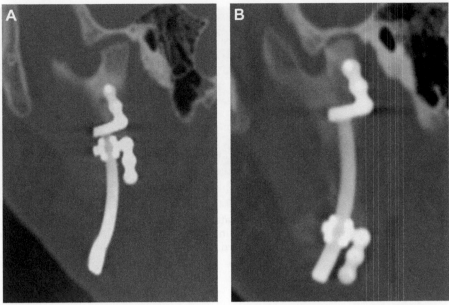

Fig. 18. Initial (*A*) and follow-up (*B*) sagittal MIP CT images show the change in position of the device for mandibular lengthening.

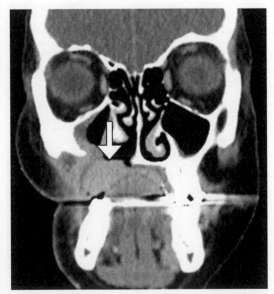

Fig. 19. Coronal CT image shows an intermediate attenuation obturator prosthesis (*arrow*) situated between the oral and sinonasal cavities status postright maxillectomy and palatectomy.

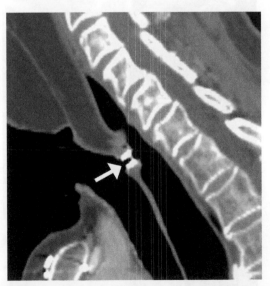

Fig. 20. Sagittal CT image shows the hyperattenuating voice prosthesis (*arrow*) that extends from the esophagus and trachea, where there is also a tracheostomy.

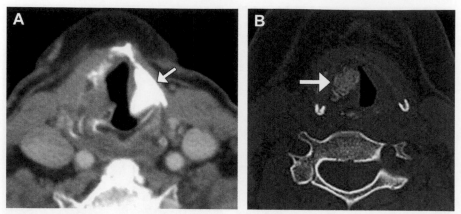

Fig. 21. Axial CT image (*A*) shows the triangular hyperattenuating silastic implant (*arrow*) in the medialized left vocal cord, which was inserted via an opening created in the thyroid cartilage. Axial CT image (*B*) shows the hyperattenuating polytetrafluoroethylene right vocal cord implant (*arrow*).

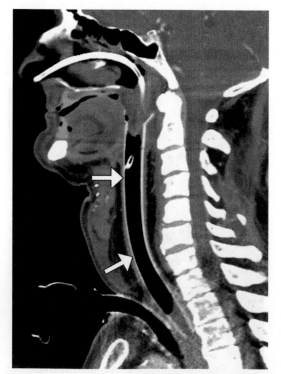

Fig. 22. Sagittal CT image shows the hyperattenuating salivary bypass tube (*arrows*) traversing the neopharynx.

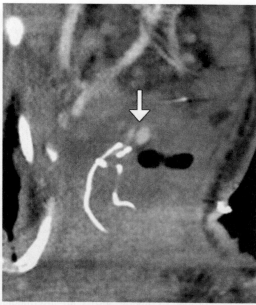

Fig. 23. Coronal CT image shows the implantable Doppler probe positioned adjacent to the vascular pedicle (*arrow*) of a soft tissue flap.

contacts and one dummy contact with an intervening lucent gap that could potentially be misconstrued as a defect in the implant on CT (**Fig. 17**).[19] In general, patients with cochlear implants can safely undergo MR imaging at 1.5 T if the device is secured, although the hardware produces considerable artifact.[20]

MANDIBULAR DISTRACTORS

Micrognathia can be treated via progressive mandibular lengthening using distraction devices.[21] The distractors are positioned across an osteotomy, and the lower part is gradually shifted down, allowing bone to grow across the gap (**Fig. 18**). Thus, the change in position of the lower segment of the distractor is an expected finding, as long as it remains affixed to the bone.

OBTURATOR PROSTHESES

Maxillectomy and palatectomy result in communications between the sinonasal and oral cavities. The defects can be closed using prostheses, which can be composed of various materials. The radiologic features of the obturator prostheses depend on the compositions and can range from air attenuation, heterogeneous, to uniformly soft tissue attenuation on CT, which can potentially mimic tumors (**Fig. 19**).[22]

TRACHEOESOPHAGEAL VOICE PROSTHESES

Voice prostheses are often used following laryngectomy and may be encountered incidentally on postoperative CT (**Fig. 20**). The devices are generally short cylindrical structures inserted across a surgically created tracheoesophageal fistula.[23] The voice prostheses are distinct from tracheostomy tubes, which may be present as well, and should not be confused with unintended retained foreign bodies. Complications related to the tracheoesophageal puncture tubes may include displacement and adjacent fistula formation, which can be evaluated via contrast swallow fluoroscopic examinations.

VOCAL CORD IMPLANTS

Vocal cord atrophy can be treated via insertion of medialization implants via thyroid cartilage windows. Various materials have been used for this purpose, including silastic implants, which appear as hyperattenuating triangular structures on axial CT images and polytetrafluoroethylene, which can appear as folded hyperattenuating strips (**Fig. 21**).[24]

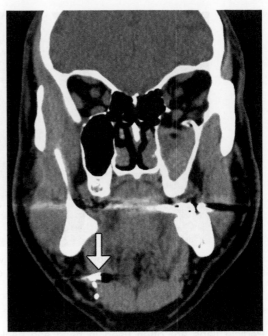

Fig. 24. Coronal CT image shows a hypoglossal nerve stimulator electrode (*arrows*) positioned in the right lateral floor of mouth.

SALIVARY BYPASS TUBES

Exposure to saliva can impair the healing of cervical esophageal and hypopharyngeal strictures and aerodigestive tract fistulae. Salivary bypass tubes have been used with the goal of preventing pharyngocutaneous fistula after laryngectomy.[25] The tubes are often composed of silicone, are flanged at the upper end, extend from the oropharynx to the esophagus, and may be encountered on routine postoperative imaging (**Fig. 22**). These tubes are secured in position, but may rarely detach and migrate through the digestive tract.

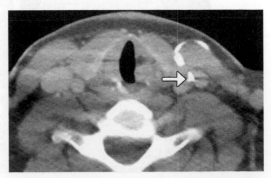

Fig. 25. Axial CT image shows the vagus nerve stimulator electrode in the left carotid space (*arrow*).

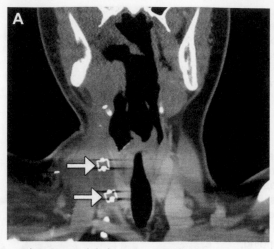

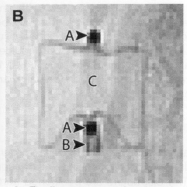

A. Radiopaque marker bands
B. Micro screw attachment
C. Nitinol mesh

Fig. 26. Coronal CT image (*A*) shows metallic basket vascular plugs (*arrows*) used to occlude the right carotid artery. Fluoroscopic image (*B*) details the components of the device.

IMPLANTABLE DOPPLER PROBE

Pedicle flaps are often used in head and neck reconstruction surgery. The viability of the flap depends on a patent vascular supply. The flaps can be salvaged if vascular compromise is promptly identified; this can be facilitated through the use of implantable Doppler probes that can monitor the adequacy of blood flow.[26] These devices appear as wiry structures that contact the vascular pedicle (**Fig. 23**).

IMPLANTABLE HYPOGLOSSAL NEUROSTIMULATOR

Electrical stimulation of the hypoglossal nerve can help maintain a patent pharyngeal airway in

patients with obstructive sleep apnea.[27] The device consists of a stimulation lead positioned in the floor of mouth (**Fig. 24**), a sensing lead, and an implantable pulse generator, which analyzes respiratory patterns and delivers stimulation synchronously with inspiration.

VAGAL NERVE STIMULATOR

Vagus nerve stimulation is performed for controlling intractable seizures.[28] The device consists of 2 electrodes and an anchor loop implanted in the left neck at the midcervical level posterolateral to the internal and common carotid arteries and medial to the internal jugular vein (**Fig. 25**). Unlike with the right vagus nerve, left vagal stimulation does not affect cardiac function. MR imaging of

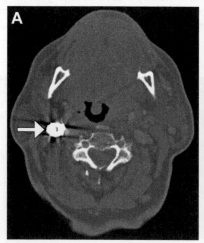

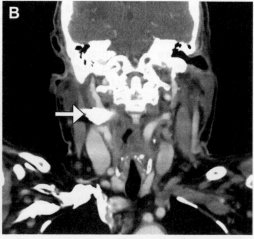

Fig. 27. Axial (*A*) and coronal (*B*) CT images show a metallic vascular clamp (*arrows*) along the course of the right carotid artery.

the brain is safe in patients with vagus nerve stimulators.[29]

VASCULAR PLUGS

Rapid endovascular vessel occlusion can be accomplished through the use of plugs.[30] These devices have a cylindrical configuration and are composed of nitinol mesh wires with identifiable radio-opaque makers on CT and fluoroscopy (**Fig. 26**). The plugs are MR imaging compatible.

VASCULAR CLAMPS

In the past, a variety of metallic vascular clamps have been used to occlude the extracranial carotid artery. As opposed to vascular plugs, these clamps have a ring-shaped configuration with an adjustable screw that is inserted around the vessel and gradually tightened (**Fig. 27**). The clamps should not be confounded with bullets or other foreign bodies, because patients with the clamps can tolerate MR imaging up to 1.5 T. In particular, ferromagnetic clamps created severe "blackhole" artifacts and image distortion on head and neck MR imaging, whereas the tantalum clips cause less artifact.[31]

SUMMARY

There is a wide variety of surgical implants and foreign bodies in the head and neck that can sometimes have confounding radiologic appearances. Familiarity with the material properties and imaging features of various materials that comprise foreign bodies and surgical implants can facilitate optimal radiological interpretation and help guide appropriate utilization of MR imaging.

CLINICS CARE POINTS

- Foreign bodies and surgical implants can sometimes be encountered incidentally on head and neck imaging performed for other reasons, but it can nevertheless be helpful to note their presence and assess for any potential complications.

- Imaging can also be specifically performed for verifying the presence or positioning of foreign bodies and surgical implants and for any associated abnormalities.

- It is helpful to be familiar with what implants or foreign bodies can safely undergo MRI and be cognizant of the associated imaging artifacts.

REFERENCES

1. McDermott M, Branstetter BF 4th, Escott EJ. What's in your mouth? The CT appearance of comestible intraoral foreign bodies. AJNR Am J Neuroradiol 2008; 29(8):1552–5.
2. Towbin AJ. The CT appearance of intraoral chewing gum. Pediatr Radiol 2008;38(12):1350–2.
3. Ho VT, McGuckin JF Jr, Smergel EM. Intraorbital wooden foreign body: CT and MR appearance. AJNR Am J Neuroradiol 1996;17(1):134-136.
4. Rong AJ, Fan KC, Golshani B, et al. Multimodal imaging features of intraocular foreign bodies. Semin Ophthalmol 2019;34(7–8):518–32.
5. Henrikson GC, Mafee MF, Flanders AE, et al. CT evaluation of plastic intraocular foreign bodies. AJNR Am J Neuroradiol 1987;8(2):378-379.
6. Radzi S, Cowin G, Robinson M, et al. Metal artifacts from titanium and steel screws in CT, 1.5T and 3T MR images of the tibial Pilon: a quantitative assessment in 3D. Quant Imaging Med Surg 2014;4(3): 163–72.
7. Schatz CJ, Ginat DT. Imaging of cosmetic facial implants and grafts. AJNR Am J Neuroradiol 2013; 34(9):1674–81.
8. Schatz CJ, Ginat DT. Imaging features of rhinoplasty. AJNR Am J Neuroradiol 2014;35(2):216–22.
9. Marra S, Leonetti JP, Konior RJ, et al. Effect of magnetic resonance imaging on implantable eyelid weights. Ann Otol Rhinol Laryngol 1995;104(6):448–52.
10. Ginat DT, Bhama P, Cunnane ME, et al. Facial reanimation procedures depicted on radiologic imaging. AJNR Am J Neuroradiol 2014;35(9):1662–6.
11. Ginat DT, Singh AD, Moonis G. Multimodality imaging of hydrogel scleral buckles. Retina 2012;32(8): 1449–52.
12. Girardot C, Hazebroucq VG, Fery-Lemonnier E, et al. MR imaging and CT of surgical materials currently used in ophthalmology: in vitro and in vivo studies. Radiology 1994;191(2):433–9.
13. Ferreira J, Fernandes F, Patricio M, et al. Magnetic resonance imaging study on blebs morphology of ahmed valves. J Curr Glaucoma Pract 2015;9(1): 1–5.
14. Mabray MC, Uzelac A, Talbott JF, et al. Ex-PRESS glaucoma filter: an MRI compatible metallic orbital foreign body imaged at 1.5 and 3T. Clin Radiol 2015;70(5):e28–34.
15. De Potter P, Duprez T, Cosnard G. Postcontrast magnetic resonance imaging assessment of porous polyethylene orbital implant (Medpor). Ophthalmology 2000;107(9):1656–60.
16. Athanasiov PA, Madge S, Kakizaki H, et al. A review of bypass tubes for proximal lacrimal drainage obstruction. Surv Ophthalmol 2011;56(3):252-266.
17. Blind A, Hulterström A, Berggren D. Treatment of nasal septal perforations with a custom-made

prosthesis. Eur Arch Otorhinolaryngol 2009;266(1): 65–9.

18. Hirsch BE, Weissman JL, Curtin HD, et al. Imaging of ossicular prostheses. Otolaryngol Head Neck Surg 1994;111(4):494–6.

19. Burck I, Drath F, Albrecht MH, et al. Visualization of different types of cochlear implants in postoperative cone-beam CT imaging. Acad Radiol 2021. S1076-6332(21)00097-0.

20. Crane BT, Gottschalk B, Kraut M, et al. Magnetic resonance imaging at 1.5 T after cochlear implantation. Otol Neurotol 2010;31(8):1215–20.

21. Sahoo NK, Issar Y, Thakral A. Mandibular distraction osteogenesis. J Craniofac Surg 2019;30(8): e743–6.

22. Kumar VA, Hofstede TM, Ginsberg LE. CT imaging features of obturator prostheses in patients following palatectomy or maxillectomy. AJNR Am J Neuroradiol 2011;32(10):1926–9.

23. Vincent ME, Robbins AH, Walsh M, et al. Evaluation of Blom-Singer voice prosthesis. AJR Am J Roentgenol 1984;143(4):745–50.

24. Vachha BA, Ginat DT, Mallur P, et al. Finding a Voice": Imaging Features after Phonosurgical Procedures for Vocal Fold Paralysis. AJNR Am J Neuroradiol 2016;37(9):1574–80.

25. Torrico Román P, García Nogales A, Trinidad Ruíz G. Utility of the Montgomery salivary tubes for preventing pharyngocutaneous fistula in total laryngectomy. Am J Otolaryngol 2020;41(4):102557.

26. Guillemaud JP, Seikaly H, Cote D, et al. The implantable Cook-Swartz Doppler probe for postoperative monitoring in head and neck free flap reconstruction. Arch Otolaryngol Head Neck Surg 2008; 134(7):729–34.

27. Maresch KJ. Hypoglossal Nerve Stimulation: Effective Longterm Therapy for Obstructive Sleep Apnea. AANA J 2018;86(5):412–6.

28. González HFJ, Yengo-Kahn A, Englot DJ. Vagus Nerve Stimulation for the Treatment of Epilepsy. Neurosurg Clin N Am 2019;30(2):219–30.

29. Benbadis SR, Nyhenhuis J, Tatum WO, et al. MRI of the brain is safe in patients implanted with the vagus nerve stimulator. Seizure 2001;10(7):512–5.

30. Banfield JC, Shankar JJ. Amplatzer vascular plug for rapid vessel occlusion in interventional neuroradiology. Interv Neuroradiol 2016;22(1):116–21.

31. Teitelbaum GP, Lin MC, Watanabe AT, et al. Ferromagnetism and MR imaging: safety of carotid vascular clamps. AJNR Am J Neuroradiol 1990; 11(2):267–72.

Skull Base Tumor Mimics

Jeffrey H. Huang, MD[a], Mari Hagiwara, MD[b],*

KEYWORDS

- Skull base • Petrous apex • Mimics

KEY POINTS

- The ability to confidently identify anatomic variants and benign pathologies that can mimic neoplasm in the skull base may help prevent unnecessary imaging follow-up, biopsies, or interventions.
- Normal variant anatomy of the central skull base includes canalis basilaris medianus, fossa navicularis magna, craniopharyngeal canal, and arrested pneumatization of the sphenoid sinus.
- Benign lesions of the central skull base include cephalocele, fibrous dysplasia, ecchordosis physaliphora, invasive or ectopic pituitary adenoma, skull base osteomyelitis, and other inflammatory processes.
- Petrous apex tumor mimics include petrous apex cephalocele, asymmetric pneumatization, petrous apex effusion, and petrous internal carotid artery aneurysm.

INTRODUCTION

The base of skull acts as a supporting structure for the brain and the primary boundary between the intracranial central nervous system and the extracranial head and neck compartments. Many different benign and malignant processes can affect the skull base, and its involvement by malignant processes can drastically alter staging, surgical approach, or radiation planning.[1–4] Clinical evaluation and tissue sampling are difficult because of its deep location, leaving imaging assessment the primary means for lesion evaluation. The purpose of this article is to familiarize readers with the imaging characteristics of various anatomic variants and benign pathologies of the skull base that can mimic more ominous pathologies, in hopes of increasing confidence of diagnosis, decreasing unnecessary procedures, and allaying patient fear.

ANATOMIC VARIANTS OF THE CENTRAL SKULL BASE

The embryologic development of the sphenoid bone is complex, with 15 separate ossification centers, containing the cephalic end of the course of the notochord, and also taking part in development of the pituitary gland.[5–8] Failure of embryologic development could produce anatomic variants including canalis basilaris medianus (CBM), fossa navicularis magna, and craniopharyngeal canal (CPC), which radiologists should be familiar with to avoid misinterpretation as pathology.

Canalis Basilaris Medianus

Anatomic variants of the basiocciput are uncommon, and the CBM, also known as the median clival canal, clival canal, or median basal canal, is one of the more well-known variants.[5,9] The CBM was first described by Gruber in 1880 and consists of a well-defined channel extending from the surface of the basiocciput.[5] Depending on the number and location of openings to the surface of the basiocciput, six different types have been described, and they are estimated to occur in about 4% to 5% of children and 2% to 3% of adults (**Fig. 1**).[5,6,9–14] These defects may close as children age, explaining the discrepancy between incidences in children and adults.

---

[a] Department of Radiology, NYU Langone Health, 462 1st Avenue, NBV-3W38, New York, NY 10016, USA;
[b] Department of Radiology, NYU Langone Health, 222 East 41st Street, 5th Floor Radiology, New York, NY 10017, USA
* Corresponding author.
E-mail address: Mari.Hagiwara@nyulangone.org

Neuroimag Clin N Am 32 (2022) 327–344
https://doi.org/10.1016/j.nic.2022.02.001

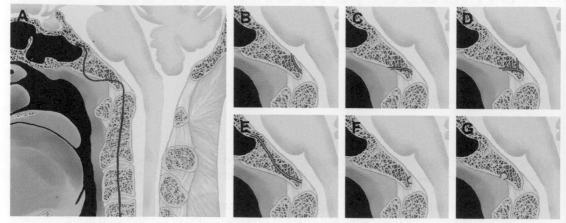

Fig. 1. Canalis basilaris medianus. The developmental notochord extends cranially to caudally through the sphenoid, sphenoccipital synchondrosis, occiput, vertebral bodies, and intervertebral disks, with a free segment in the nasopharynx (*A*). CBM complete types include superior (*B*), inferior (*C*), and bifurcatus (*D*). CBM incomplete types include long-channel (*E*), superior recess (*F*), and inferior recess (*G*).

Three types of complete CBM have been described. The superior type exhibits a superior inferior channel through the clivus connecting two openings on the dorsal aspect of the basiocciput. The inferior type exhibits an anterior-posterior channel connecting openings on the dorsal and ventral aspects of the basiocciput. The bifurcatus type exhibits a bifurcated channel connecting two openings on the dorsal aspect and one opening on the ventral aspect of the basiocciput.

Three types of incomplete CBM have been described. The long-channel type exhibits a long channel extending from the dorsal aspect of the basiocciput toward the basisphenoid. The superior and inferior recess types exhibit round defects along the dorsal and ventral aspects of the basiocciput (see **Fig. 1**).

On imaging, the complete types or the incomplete long channel type appear as 1- to 2-mm wide, well-corticated, midline, channel-like defects extending from the dorsal aspect of the basiocciput (**Fig. 2**). The incomplete recess types appear as round, well-corticated midline defects along the surface of the basiocciput and may contain adenoid lymphoid tissue in the case of the inferior recess type, which is misinterpreted as a mass. The longitudinal extent of the CBM may be more easily assessed on thin-slice sagittal computed tomography (CT) images.

There are two main theories explaining the development of the CBM.[5,6,15] The first is that the CBM is simply a vascular channel containing venous structures (emissary veins) connecting to the basilar venous plexus. A few studies have demonstrated only the presence of vascular structures within the canal.[9,14] The second, more likely theory is that the CBM represents remnant notochordal tissue. In utero, the notochord courses within the vertebral bodies caudally. Cranially, the notochord courses within the basiocciput and ends in the posterior sphenoid, with a free segment within the pharyngeal wall ventral to the clivus.[5,6,15] The notochord is enclosed by the osseous structures and degenerates, leaving remnants within the clivus and nucleus pulposi.[6,15] Failure of different portions of the notochordal canal to close entirely is thought to result in the CBM.

Although the CBM is generally thought to be a benign anatomic variant, there have been case reports of potentially related complications. Nguyen and colleagues[16] reported a case of a nasopharyngeal chordoma associated with a CBM, which also lends credence to the theory that the CBM represents remnant notochordal tissue. Additional potential complications include basioccipital meningocele, recurrent meningitis, pharyngeal enterogenous cysts, nasopharyngeal Tornwaldt cysts, and cerebrospinal fluid (CSF) leaks.[6,17–22]

Fossa Navicularis Magna

The fossa navicularis magna, also known as the fossa pharyngea, large pharyngeal fossa, keyhole defect, CBM, and longitudinal or transverse segmentations, is another anatomic variant of the ventral aspect of the basiocciput.[5,23,24] It is estimated to occur in approximately 1% to 8% of the population, without any significant difference in incidence between males and females.[11,25–27]

On imaging, the fossa navicularis magna appears as a well-defined, well-corticated, notchlike midline defect along the ventral aspect of the clivus and contains soft tissue (**Fig. 3**), similar in

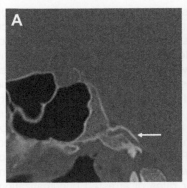
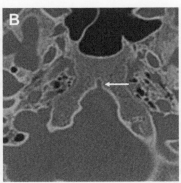
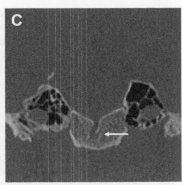

Fig. 2. Incomplete long channel type canalis basilaris medianus. Sagittal (A), axial (B), and coronal (C) computed tomography images demonstrate a long, thin, well-corticated, channel-like midline osseous defect in the dorsal surface of the clivus, extending from the dorsal aspect of the basiocciput toward the basisphenoid (arrows). (Courtesy of G. Moonis, MD, New York, New York).

appearance to the inferior recess type CBM.[5,23,24,28] It can appear as a keyhole-shaped defect, with a narrow neck extending to a deep larger round defect. It may contain lymphoid tissue from the nasopharyngeal adenoids.[24] At the bottom of the fossa navicularis, there may be a round or ovoid recess, called the pharyngeal fossa.[5,28]

Given the similarity of its appearance, the fossa navicularis magna may actually represent the inferior recess variant of an incomplete CBM.[5,23,28] It is also thought to represent remnant notochordal tissue, rather than prominent emissary veins.[5,29]

The fossa navicularis magna is generally thought to be a benign anatomic variant, but it may occasionally serve as a route of spread for infection via primary infection or abscess formation within the lymphoid tissue of the fossa navicularis, resulting in clival osteomyelitis and intracranial spread.[11,28–31]

Craniopharyngeal Canal

The CPC, also known as the persistent CPC, persistent hypophyseal canal, or transsphenoidal canal, is another skull base anatomic variant,

appearing as a well-corticated, midline, linear defect of the sphenoid, extending from the floor of the sella turcica to the nasopharynx.[7,8,32,33] It is rare, occurring in approximately 0.3% to 0.4% of the population, and larger defects may actually reflect meningoencephaloceles related to dysraphism and occur with other midline craniofacial abnormalities, such as optic apparatus abnormalities, agenesis of the corpus callosum, PHACES syndrome, cleft lip, or cleft palate.[11,32–34]

The pituitary gland is formed by fusion of Rathke pouch, which forms as a diverticulum from the roof of the stomodeum migrating superiorly, with the floor of the diencephalon migrating inferiorly.[8] The presphenoid and postsphenoid cartilages then fuse, resulting in closure of Rathke pouch. Failure of the cartilage to fuse leaves behind a residual canal, the CPC.[7,8,32,33] Remnant pituitary tissue has been found within a CPC, supporting this theory.[35]

Although the CPC is a benign variant, its presence may have important clinical and surgical implications. A large CPC may be lined by dura that joins with the periosteum on the undersurface of the sphenoid, resulting in CSF leaks or recurrent

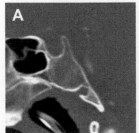
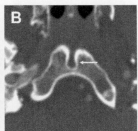
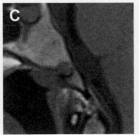
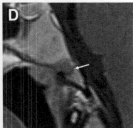

Fig. 3. Fossa navicularis. Sagittal CT image (A) shows a round, well-corticated osseous notchlike midline defect in the ventral surface of the clivus containing soft tissue. Axial CT image (B) shows the defect is midline, with a keyhole configuration (arrow). Noncontrast (C) and contrast-enhanced (D) T1-weighted (T1W) MR images show the soft tissue within the fossa is continuous with and enhances similarly to the nasopharyngeal tissues, reflecting adenoidal lymphoid tissue (arrow).

meningitis.[33,36–40] The pituitary gland itself may herniate through the canal and the canal may be associated with masses, such as pituitary adenomas, craniopharyngiomas, dermoids, and nasopharyngeal gliomas (heterotopic neuroglial tissue), which is mistaken for skull base or primary nasopharyngeal polyps or neoplasm. Pituitary tissue may be inadvertently resected during surgery, resulting in iatrogenic hypopituitarism or CSF leak.[7,8,32,41–44]

In 2014, Abele and colleagues[8] proposed a classification system composed of three main types of CPC. Type 1 is described as a small incidental canal (Fig. 4), type 2 as a medium-sized canal containing ectopic adenohypophysis, type 3A as a large canal with associated cephalocele, type 3B as a large canal with associated tumors of the adenohypophysis or associated embryonic tissues (Fig. 5), and type 3C as a large canal with associated tumors of both tissue types. Type 2 and type 3 CPC may be associated with higher rates of pituitary dysfunction, and type 3 CPC may be more prone to surgical complications, such as iatrogenic hypopituitarism or CSF leak.

Arrested Pneumatization of the Sphenoid Sinus

Pneumatization of the paranasal sinuses begins in utero, with maturation continuing through the third decade of life.[45–49] Alteration of this process can result in hypoplastic, aplastic, or accessory sinuses. Arrested pneumatization, most frequently involving the sphenoid sinus, is a developmental variant with imaging features that may be easily confused with more concerning pathologies.[45,50,51]

At birth, the sphenoid bones contain erythropoietic marrow, which undergoes yellow fatty marrow conversion within the presphenoid plate starting before 2 years of age.[45–48] The process extends posteriorly into the basisphenoid. Conversion here precedes the normal marrow conversion of the clivus.[45] Respiratory mucosa extends into the areas of yellow marrow and results in pneumatization as early as 2 years of age and extends to the sphenoccipital synchondrosis, attaining maturity by 14 to 16 years.[45–49] Marrow conversion is thought to be triggered by changes in blood supply or oxygenation, but it is not clearly understood.[48,52] Patients with sickle cell or thalassemia, with diseased red blood cells, seem to have higher rates of arrested pneumatization, lending credence to this idea.[51]

When arrested pneumatization occurs, atypical fatty marrow persists within the sphenoid bone adjacent to the aerated sinuses, most commonly in expected regions of normal or accessory sphenoid sinus pneumatization. These locations include the basisphenoid, pterygoid processes, and clivus.[45] On CT, it appears as a well-circumscribed, nonexpansile lesion with well-corticated margins and varying amounts of internal fat and internal curvilinear calcifications.[45] On MR imaging, it appears as a lesion with higher T1 signal than that of surrounding normal bone marrow (Fig. 6) and may have subtle patchy enhancement.[45] Given its imaging features, it may be misinterpreted as chordoma, chondrosarcoma, fibrous dysplasia (FD), osteomyelitis, or metastatic disease and can lead to unnecessary imaging, biopsy, or treatment.[45,50]

To allow for more confident diagnosis of arrested pneumatization, Welker and colleagues[45] in 2008 proposed a set of diagnostic criteria: (1) location at a site of normal or accessory pneumatization; (2) nonexpansile lesion with sclerotic, well-circumscribed margins; and (3) demonstrating fat content, internal curvilinear

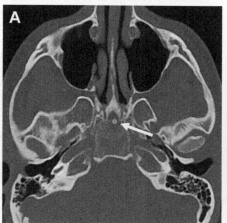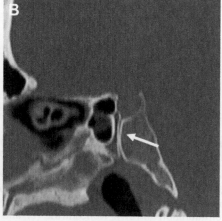

Fig. 4. Type 1 CPC. Axial (*A*) and sagittal (*B*) CT images show a narrow, well-corticated, midline channel through the clivus, extending from the floor of the sella turcica to the roof of the nasopharynx (*arrows*).

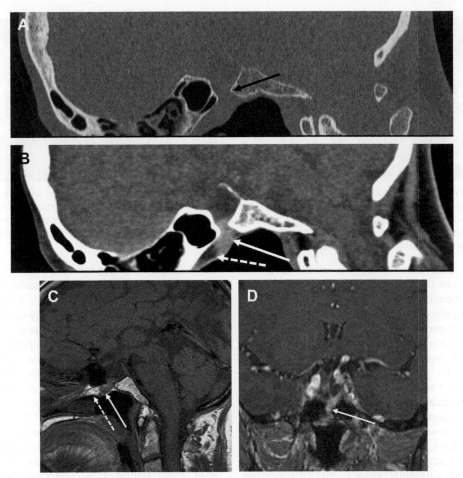

Fig. 5. Type 3B CPC. Sagittal CT images in bone (*A*) and soft tissue (*B*) windows show a large well-corticated craniopharyngeal canal/defect (*black arrow*) in the floor of the sella turcica, with herniated pituitary tissue (*white arrow*) and a fat-containing lesion anteriorly, likely a dermoid (*dashed arrow*). Sagittal precontrast (*C*) and coronal postcontrast (*D*) T1W MR images show the enhancing herniated pituitary tissue (*solid arrows*) and T1 hyperintense dermoid (*dashed arrow*).

calcifications, and normal appearance of any associated skull base foramina.

BENIGN LESIONS
Cephalocele

Cephaloceles are an extension or protrusion of any intracranial contents through a defect of the cranium and dura mater.[53–55] When they contain herniated brain tissue, they are termed encephaloceles. Congenital cephaloceles are rare, with an incidence of approximately 0.8 to 4 per 10,000 live births. They are thought to represent a primary anomaly of formation and separation of the neural tube from the body surface. As a result, they occur in conjunction with other intracranial and extracranial developmental anomalies in up to 50%.[53–60] These more commonly occur posteriorly (occipital or parietal) than anteriorly (frontoethmoidal),[54–56] and they are most often

midline but can occur off midline, such as into the paranasal sinuses or petrous apices.[53,61,62]

Acquired cephaloceles can occur as a result of prior trauma, surgery, tumors, sphenoid dysplasia, or osteoradionecrosis, or they are spontaneous. Spontaneous cephaloceles are often seen in obese middle-aged women with idiopathic intracranial hypertension, where the increased intracranial pressure, associated prominent arachnoid granulations, and progressive bony thinning are thought to lead to CSF leaks and herniation of the dura or brain.[63] Spontaneous cephaloceles and CSF leaks are typically seen in areas of thin bone including the cribriform plates, areas bordering the pneumatized paranasal sinuses, and the tegmen tympani.[63]

Imaging demonstrates a sac of fluid with or without brain tissue extending from the intracranial compartment through an osseous defect, with CT best demonstrating the bony defect and MR

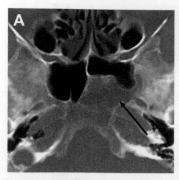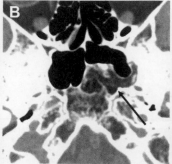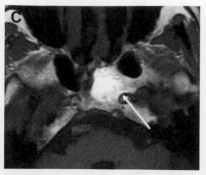

Fig. 6. Arrested pneumatization of the left sphenoid sinus. Axial CT images in bone (A) and soft tissue (B) windows show a well-circumscribed, well-corticated, lesion with internal curvilinear calcifications centered on a normal area of sphenoid pneumatization in the left sphenoid body (*arrows*). Soft tissue window demonstrates central fat density. Axial T1W MR image (C) shows the lesion demonstrates higher signal than the adjacent normal marrow within the clivus and sphenoid.

imaging best determining the contents of the cephalocele (Fig. 7). The sac and brain tissue may demonstrate heterogeneous enhancement. Cisternogram with intrathecal contrast administration may demonstrate leakage of contrast into the sac or into the surrounding tissues, as in the case of a CSF leak. On imaging, cephaloceles are mistaken for cystic or solid masses, therefore attention for skull base defects should be made for lesions bordering the skull base.

Cephaloceles can herniate into the paranasal sinuses, where they may be mistaken for mucoceles, polyps, or primary neoplasms on imaging and endoscopically.[62] When herniating into sinuses, they frequently present with CSF rhinorrhea but can also present with recurrent meningitis or, if large enough, airway obstruction.[53,62] Accurate diagnosis of cephaloceles is important because biopsy or resection runs a risk of iatrogenic intracranial infections, parenchymal contusion, or CSF leaks.[53] Surgical goals for these patients may include removal of the sac and any dysplastic brain tissue, preservation of any normal brain tissue, and secure closure of the wound.[56,57]

Fibrous Dysplasia

FD is a benign, slowly progressing, dysplastic process affecting osteogenesis, characterized by the replacement of normal medullary bone with abnormal fibrous tissue interspersed with irregularly shaped trabeculae of woven bone on histology.[64–67] It is thought to be caused by an activating missense mutation of the GNAS gene on chromosome 20, affecting the Gs protein alpha subunit and resulting in increased cAMP levels.[65,67,68] This mutation is seen in the areas of abnormal bone and in patients with McCune-Albright syndrome.

FD accounts for approximately 5% to 10% of all osseous tumors and has been classified with three main forms: (1) monostotic (80%); (2) polyostotic (20%); and (3) McCune-Albright syndrome, which is polyostotic disease with endocrine dysfunction, abnormal skin pigmentation, and precocious puberty.[64,65,67,68] Polyostotic disease can also be seen with other disorders, including primary hyperparathyroidism, tuberous sclerosis, and Mazabraud syndrome.[65,68] FD most commonly affects the craniofacial bones, in 10% to 25% of cases of monostotic disease and 50% to 100% of cases of polyostotic disease, predominantly affecting the ethmoid (71%), followed by the sphenoid (43%), frontal (33%), and maxilla (29%), with temporal bone involvement being rare.[67–70] Most patients with the disorder are asymptomatic, but presenting symptoms are usually related to the site of disease, such as facial asymmetry, sinusitis, vision loss from optic canal involvement, headache, hearing loss from temporal bone involvement, or facial pain.[65,67,69]

Imaging features of FD are variable and confusing. On CT, the intramedullary lesions are described as well-defined and expansile, with internal "ground-glass" density, cortical thinning, and endosteal scalloping, although lesions may also appear completely lucent or sclerotic. MR imaging features are nonspecific and depend on the amount of fibrous tissue present within the abnormal bone. They typically demonstrate intermediate signal intensity but may show higher T2 signal in lesions with less osseous trabeculation or more cystic change.[65,68] Lesions are highly vascular and can enhance intensely. Given the enhancement and variable MR imaging features, FD is often mistaken for skull base neoplasm on MR imaging. When MR imaging evaluation is equivocal, CT imaging may be helpful to evaluate for the characteristic internal "ground-glass" density (Fig. 8).

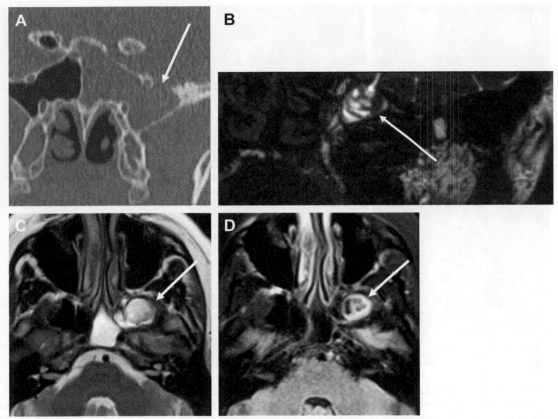

Fig. 7. Left greater sphenoid wing encephalocele. Coronal (*A*) CT image shows an osseous defect (*arrow*) through the left greater sphenoid wing with complete opacification of the left sphenoid sinus. Sagittal T2 SPACE (*B*), axial T2W (*C*), and axial contrast-enhanced T1W (*D*) MR images show abnormally enhancing herniated dysplastic, gliotic brain tissue extending from the adjacent temporal lobe into the left sphenoid sinus (*arrows*).

Imaging is clinically useful for evaluating for extent of disease and for rare complications of FD, including associated aneurysmal bone cyst formation, impingement on the optic nerve or temporal bone structures, and malignant degeneration.[65–69] Rapid expansion of the lesion, associated pain, bone destruction, or soft tissue invasion should raise suspicion for malignant degeneration, which occurs most commonly as osteosarcoma, fibrosarcoma, chondrosarcoma, or malignant fibrous histiocytosis.[65,66]

Ecchordosis Physaliphora

Ecchordosis physaliphora (EP) is a small, gelatinous benign, hamartomatous mass derived from remnant notochordal tissue, usually at midline along the dorsal wall of the clivus or in the sacrococcygeal region, although they can occur anywhere along the route of the notochord.[71–76]

EP are usually asymptomatic and found in 0.4% to 2.0% of autopsies.[72–78] They are usually intradural at the level of Dorello canal, attached to the dorsal wall of the clivus by an osseous stalk or pedicle. This contrasts with the related, rarer chordoma, a malignant neoplasm derived from notochordal remnant tissue, which is typically symptomatic, aggressive, and intraosseous, constituting 2% to 4% of primary bone tumors.[71,72,78] There have been case reports, however, of symptomatic EP with CSF fistulas into the sphenoid sinus, cervical spine EP resulting in hemiparesis and hemihypoesthesia, spontaneous pneumocephalus and pneumoventricle, headache, abducens nerve palsy, intracranial hypertension, intratumoral hemorrhage, CSF rhinorrhea, meningitis, and spontaneous rupture resulting in recurrent pneumocephalus and presenting as imbalance, headache, and rhinorrhea.[77,79–86]

Regarding imaging features of EP, CT imaging is generally limited and may only be useful for assessing for an associated osseous stalk arising from the clivus or confirming smooth well-defined bony margins. MR imaging is more helpful, with EP typically appearing as a homogeneous, T1 hypointense, T2 hyperintense, well-circumscribed, midline mass along the dorsal wall of the clivus (**Fig. 9**).[72–75,77,79] Given the

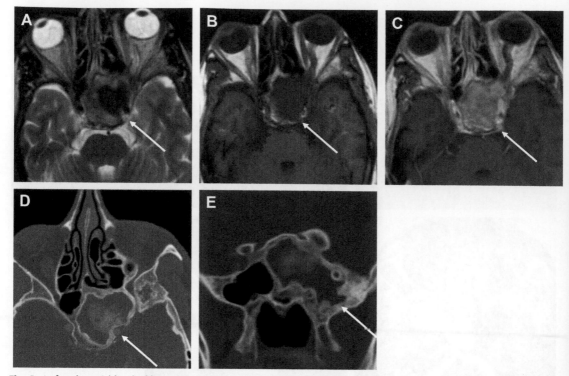

Fig. 8. Left sphenoid body fibrous dysplasia. Axial T2W (*A*), T1W (*B*), and T1W contrast-enhanced (*C*) MR images demonstrate a lobulated T2 heterogeneous, T1 hypointense, enhancing lesion in the left sphenoid body (*arrows*). The MR imaging appearance mimics a malignant neoplasm. Axial (*D*) and coronal (*E*) CT images demonstrate an expansile lesion with preservation of the cortices and internal ground-glass density (*arrows*) compatible with fibrous dysplasia. Note the predominant lucent component, which can be seen with fibrous dysplasia.

location and signal characteristics of EP, it can be mistaken for lesions such as chordoma, chondrosarcoma, or metastasis, but EP should not demonstrate any aggressive, bony destructive features. EP typically also does not demonstrate contrast enhancement, whereas chordoma typically avidly enhances.[72–75,77,78,83] Any bony destruction, inhomogeneous signal characteristics, loculations, or contrast enhancement should raise suspicion for a malignant pathology. There have been case reports of enhancing EP and nonenhancing chordoma, however, so contrast enhancement characteristics are not entirely reliable, and imaging follow-up is generally recommended.[74]

Invasive and Ectopic Pituitary Adenoma

Pituitary adenomas are the most common lesions found in the sella turcica and among the most common primary brain tumors overall, accounting for 10% to 15% of primary brain tumors.[87,88] Most pituitary adenomas remain confined to the sellar space, but large invasive pituitary adenomas (IPA) may demonstrate extrasellar extension, often extending into the suprasellar space or cavernous sinuses.[89–92] Uncommonly, large pituitary adenomas can demonstrate infrasellar extension,

involving the clivus, sphenoid sinus, and even the pharynx, petrosal sinus, jugular foramen, or hypoglossal canal.[87,88,90,92–94] Given the location and invasive features of the IPA, these lesions are mistaken for more aggressive skull base neoplasms, such as chordoma, chondrosarcoma, meningioma, astrocytoma, craniopharyngioma, or metastases.[87,88,93]

Pituitary adenomas may also rarely be ectopic in location and can arise anywhere along the course of Rathke pouch as it extends to the sella turcica in utero.[87,88,95,96] They are most common in the sphenoid sinus, although they are also seen in the nasopharynx, cavernous sinus, and uncommonly in the clivus. When occurring in the skull base or other ectopic locations, these can also be mistaken for neoplasm.

On imaging, IPA typically demonstrates smooth enlargement of the sella turcica and when invading the cavernous sinus, it typically encases the cavernous internal carotid artery (ICA) without associated vascular narrowing (**Fig. 10**). Various imaging features may help to differentiate pituitary adenoma from malignant neoplasms, such as lower T2 signal, more avid enhancement, and lower apparent diffusion coefficient of IPA when

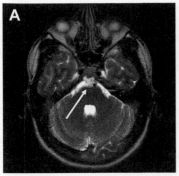
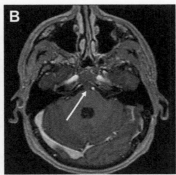
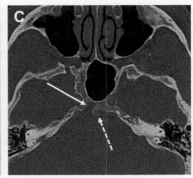

Fig. 9. Ecchordosis physaliphora. Axial T2W (A) and T1W contrast-enhanced (B) MR images show a small, well-circumscribed, nonenhancing lesion within the dorsal clivus extending into the prepontine cistern (arrows). Axial CT image (C) in a different patient demonstrates a well-defined lobulated defect in the right aspect of the clivus (solid arrow) with an osseous stalk extending posteriorly from the midline clivus (dashed arrow).

compared with chordoma and other malignant processes.[93] Atypical features for IPA, such as enlargement of the pituitary stalk, rapid growth, clival or sellar destruction, or luminal narrowing of the ICA when cavernous sinus invasion is present, should point away from IPA.[97] Sellar enlargement occurs in nearly 100% of pituitary macroadenomas, and although it is also seen in nonadenomatous masses, its absence, or the presence of erosion without enlargement, is suggestive of other neoplasms.[98]

Skull Base Osteomyelitis and Inflammatory Processes

Given the complexity of the skull base and its surrounding structures, there are a multitude of infectious and inflammatory processes that can present with confusing clinical and imaging characteristics. For example, inflammatory pseudotumor (IPT), granulomatosis with polyangiitis, sarcoidosis, IgG4-related sclerosing disease, osteomyelitis, fungal sinusitis, and Langerhans cell histiocytosis may all have varied and nonspecific clinical and imaging findings, creating diagnostic

difficulty and often requiring biopsy to differentiate them from chordoma, chondrosarcoma, nasopharyngeal carcinoma, or metastases.[99]

Skull base osteomyelitis (SBO) involving the cranial vault or skull base is rare, with the incidence of SBO higher in developing countries, thought likely to be related to lower antibiotic use.[100–103] Recent history of an otogenic or sinonasal infection, fever, or leukocytosis in at-risk elderly patients with diabetes or immunocompromised patients can help suggest this diagnosis.[100,101,103] Symptoms, however, may be nonspecific, with an insidious and delayed onset of symptoms, such as headache and facial pain, with presentation starting many weeks after resolution of an initial otogenic or sinonasal infection.[101–103] This can lead to delays in diagnosis, and diagnosis might only be made after onset of neurologic deficits from cranial nerve involvement or compression, which carries a worse prognosis.[102,103]

On imaging, SBO may appear as a soft tissue mass with bone erosion or demineralization and inflammatory changes on CT, although it is often occult in its early stages. MR imaging is more

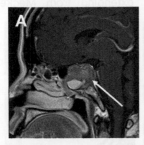
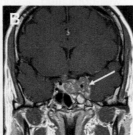
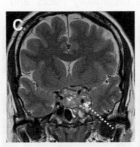
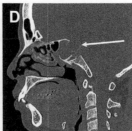

Fig. 10. Invasive pituitary adenoma. Sagittal (A) contrast-enhanced MR image demonstrates a heterogeneously enhancing mass (arrow) in the central skull base with no identifiable separate pituitary tissue. Coronal contrast-enhanced T1W (B) and T2W (C) MR images demonstrate invasion of the left cavernous sinus (solid arrow) and encasement of the cavernous left ICA (dashed arrow), without associated vascular narrowing, characteristic for a pituitary adenoma. Sagittal CT image (D) demonstrates smooth remodeling and expansion of the central skull base by the adenoma (arrow).

useful for evaluating the extent of the disease, appearing as an infiltrative, hypointense mass on T1-weighted (T1W) images that demonstrates contrast enhancement and surrounding inflammation (Fig. 11). It demonstrates variable signal intensity on T2-weighted (T2W) images, with hypointense signal thought to be related to the chronicity of the inflammatory process and the degree of fibrosis.[102,103] SBO may demonstrate reduced diffusion, particularly in areas of abscess formation.[104] Delayed diagnosis of SBO can also lead to complications, such as intracranial spread, arterial involvement and infarct, pseudoaneurysm, and venous sinus thrombosis.[101] Biopsy is often necessary to guide treatment, because SBO may be treated with long-term antibiotics or conservative surgery, differing from inflammatory or malignant processes.[100]

IPT, also known as plasma cell granuloma or myofibroblastic pseudotumor, is a benign, inflammatory process demonstrating acute and chronic inflammatory cells and fibrosis on histopathology.[105,106] Many patients also exhibit elevated serum IgG4 levels and IgG4-positive plasma cells on pathology, suggesting that some IPT may reflect a manifestation of IgG4-related sclerosing disease.[105,107,108] Although it most commonly occurs in the orbit, it can involve other areas, including the brain, cavernous sinus, nasopharynx, and skull base.[105,106,109] On MR imaging, it appears as an infiltrative enhancing mass; marked T2 hypointensity is suggestive of IPT and other chronic inflammatory processes. MR imaging can help evaluate for cranial nerve compression or involvement, which can result in cranial nerve palsies, pain, vision changes, or hearing loss.[105–110] IPT is generally treated with steroids and/or radiation therapy.[105]

Granulomatosis with polyangiitis is an autoimmune vasculitis involving small and medium sized vessels, characterized by necrotizing granulomatous inflammation of the respiratory tracts and necrotizing glomerulonephritis.[111] Although granulomatosis with polyangiitis is thought of as a disease of the respiratory tracts and kidneys that can spread systemically to involve any organ, 10% of patients present initially with isolated skull base disease causing cranial neuropathies.[111–113] It may appear as a diffuse, infiltrative enhancing mass involving the skull base and surrounding soft tissues; like IPT, marked T2W hypointensity can suggest a chronic inflammatory process not typically seen with neoplasm (Fig. 12). Clinical history, laboratory evaluation of serum antineutrophil cytoplasmic antibodies, and possibly tissue sampling are key for accurate diagnosis and appropriate treatment. Treatment may involve steroids or cytotoxic agents.[112–114]

PETROUS APEX

The petrous apex is a small region of the skull base with complex anatomy, lending itself to involvement by a variety of different pathologies.[115–117] Petrous apex lesions are generally characterized as operative (neoplastic or inflammatory) or nonoperative (incidental), with most nonneoplastic lesions occurring as a result of air cell disease, such as cholesterol granuloma, cholesteatoma, or mucocele.[115] The petrous apex is difficult to clinically evaluate because of its depth, thus imaging is important for differentiation between operative and nonoperative lesions to guide management.

Petrous Apex Cephalocele

Petrous apex cephalocele (PAC) is a rare congenital or acquired lesion characterized by herniation of dura mater or arachnoid from the posterolateral portion of Meckel cave into the anterior petrous apex.[115–117] It may reflect a meningocele or arachnoid cyst. On CT, it appears as a homogeneously hypoattenuating, fluid density, circumscribed, well-corticated lesion extending from Meckel

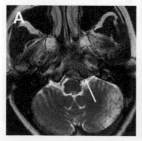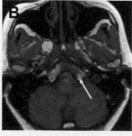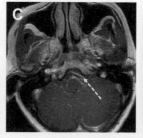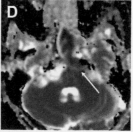

Fig. 11. Skull base osteomyelitis arising from sphenoid sinusitis. Axial T2W (*A*) and T1W (*B*) MR images show ill-defined hypointensity within the clivus (*arrows*). Axial contrast-enhanced T1W MR image (*C*) shows enhancement of the area and leptomeningeal enhancement and rim enhancement around an epidural abscess, reflecting intracranial spread (*dashed arrow*). Apparent diffusion coefficient map (*D*) shows reduced diffusion within the affected skull base and the epidural collection (*arrow*).

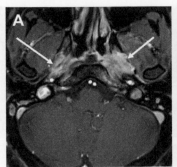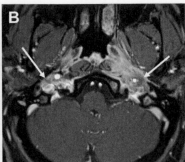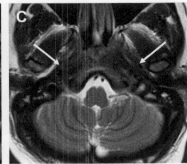

Fig. 12. Skull base granulomatosis with polyangiitis. Axial contrast-enhanced T1W fat-saturated (*A* and *B*) and T2W (*C*) MR images demonstrate ill-defined enhancement in the left greater than right parapharyngeal and carotid spaces (*arrows*), clivus, and surrounding soft tissues. Note the marked hypointense signal on T2W images suggesting chronic inflammatory tissue.

cave and eroding into the anterior petrous apex.[115–117] On MR imaging, it follows fluid signal and can contain traversing trigeminal nerve fibers (**Figs. 13** and **14**). They may have a mildly enhancing thin wall, but they do not demonstrate reduced diffusion.[115,117]

Most PACs are asymptomatic and incidentally found, but when symptomatic they may present with headache, CSF rhinorrhea, CSF leak, trigeminal neuralgia, or symptoms of intracranial hypertension.[115,117] They are usually unilateral, but can be bilateral.[61,115,117] The exact cause of PAC is not definitely known, but it may be caused by altered CSF dynamics resulting in intracranial hypertension, with herniation of the meninges into the petrous apex occurring as a natural pathway to alleviate pressure.[115,117] This is supported by

the association of PAC with symptoms of intracranial hypertension and with imaging evidence of empty sella in up to 69%.[117]

Asymmetric Pneumatization of the Petrous Apex

Although most petrous apices are filled with normal fatty marrow, they are pneumatized in up to 35%.[118,119] Pneumatization of the petrous apices is usually bilateral and symmetric but is asymmetric in 4%.[118,120] When the petrous apices are asymmetrically pneumatized, with one non-pneumatized or underpneumatized, the normal high signal of the marrow on T1W images of the nonpneumatized petrous apex is mistaken for cholesterol granulomas or misinterpreted as enhancement.[118] It does, however, suppress on

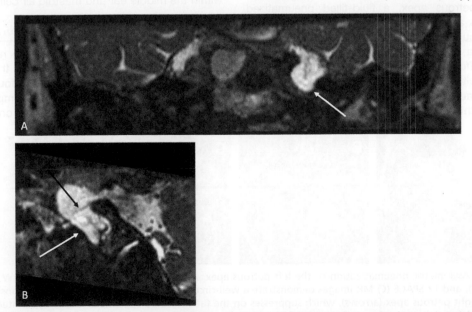

Fig. 13. Left petrous apex cephalocele. Coronal (*A*) and sagittal (*B*) T2 SPACE MR images show a circumscribed left petrous apex cephalocele extending from the posterior aspect of Meckel cave into the left petrous apex (*white arrows*). There are traversing trigeminal nerve fibers extending into the cephalocele (*black arrow*).

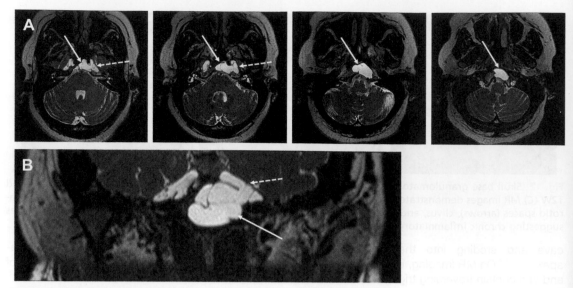

Fig. 14. Left petrous apex cephalocele. Axial (*A*) and coronal (*B*) T2 SPACE MR images demonstrate a homogeneous, well-circumscribed, lesion following CSF signal in the petrous apex and clivus (*solid arrows*), continuous with the inferior aspect of the left Meckel cave (*dashed arrows*). This was initially misinterpreted as a skull base neoplasm.

fat-suppressed imaging and it does not expand the petrous apex or exhibit reduced diffusion.[116,118,120] CT imaging can further elucidate the diagnosis by demonstrating normal marrow and cortex of the nonpneumatized petrous apex (**Fig. 15**).

Petrous Apex Effusion

In addition to misinterpretation of the nonpneumatized petrous apex, a fluid-filled pneumatized petrous apex may also be mistaken for pathologies, such as petrous apicitis, congenital cholesteatoma, cholesterol granuloma, or tumor. Petrous apex effusions appear hyperintense on T2W images, with variable signal on T1W images thought to be caused by variable amounts of protein content within the trapped fluid, with preservation of

the bony septations and cortex on CT (**Fig. 16**).[119,121,122] Cholesterol granulomas, in contrast, present symptomatically with intrinsic T1 hyperintensity on MR imaging and bony expansion and loss of the normal osseous trabeculae/septations on CT images (**Fig. 17**).[119,122] Patients with petrous apicitis also usually present symptomatically, and imaging demonstrates surrounding inflammation, osseous erosions, and fluid within the middle ear and mastoid air cells.[118]

Petrous Internal Carotid Artery Aneurysm

Aneurysms of the extradural ICA are rare, and aneurysms of the petrous segment of the extradural ICA are extremely rare, usually found incidentally.[123–127] When patients are symptomatic from petrous ICA aneurysms, they commonly

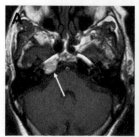
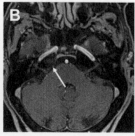
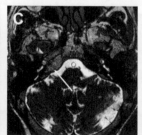
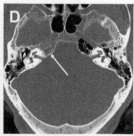

Fig. 15. Asymmetric pneumatization of the left petrous apex. Axial T1W (*A*), contrast-enhanced T1W fat-saturated (*B*), and T2 SPACE (*C*) MR images demonstrate a well-circumscribed, T1 hyperintense, nonexpansile lesion in the right petrous apex (*arrows*), which suppresses on the fat-saturated sequence. The T1 hyperintensity was confused for a cholesterol granuloma. Axial CT image (*D*) demonstrates normal marrow characteristics in the right petrous apex (*arrow*), appearing similar to the adjacent clivus, with preservation of the cortex, and a pneumatized left petrous apex.

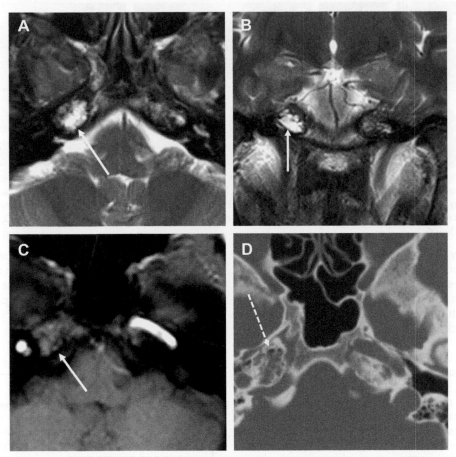

Fig. 16. Right petrous apex effusion. Axial (*A*) and coronal (*B*) T2W MR images show T2 hyperintense signal within the right petrous apex (*arrows*). Axial T1W MR image (*C*) shows corresponding intermediate to hyperintense signal (*arrow*). A follow-up axial CT image (*D*) shows a pneumatized right petrous apex with fluid, with preservation of the septations and cortex. There are a few foci of antidependent air along the anterior portion of the petrous apex (*dashed arrow*).

present with cranial nerve symptoms resulting from mass effect of the aneurysm, but they may also present with headache, Horner syndrome, pulsatile tinnitus, sensorineural hearing loss, thromboembolic events, cavernous sinus syndrome, or life-threatening otorrhagia or epistaxis.[123–125,128–131]

On CT, they appear as slightly hyperattenuating masses expanding and scalloping the petrous apex. They may also exhibit peripheral thrombus or wall calcifications. On MR imaging, they may exhibit a variety of appearances depending on the presence of thrombus, slow flow, or turbulent flow. If the aneurysm has a significant amount of

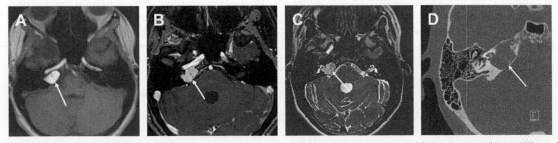

Fig. 17. Right petrous apex cholesterol granuloma. Axial T1W (*A*), contrast-enhanced fat-suppressed T1W (*B*), and T2 SPACE (*C*) MR images demonstrate a well-circumscribed, homogeneous, intrinsically T1 hyperintense lesion in the right petrous apex without obvious enhancement (*arrow*). Axial CT image (*D*) demonstrates a lucent, expansile, well-circumscribed lesion (*arrow*) with loss of the central septations.

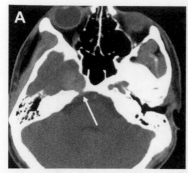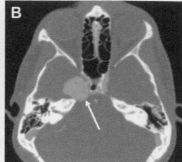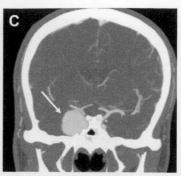

Fig. 18. Right petrous ICA aneurysm. Axial noncontrast CT image (*A*) and axial (*B*) and coronal (*C*) maximum intensity projection CT angiogram images demonstrate a hyperdense, well-circumscribed, homogeneous, arterially enhancing saccular outpouching (*arrows*) arising from the petrous ICA and extending superiorly through a defect in the petrous part of the temporal bone into the middle cranial fossa. (*Courtesy of* G. Moonis, MD, New York, New York).

flow, they may demonstrate a flow void within the central portion of the aneurysm. Turbulent flow may appear as more heterogeneous, intermediate signal on T1W and T2W images, and slow flow or thrombosis may appear as a soft tissue mass and demonstrate homogeneous enhancement.[116,123,124] Given the varied imaging characteristics, these can be mistaken for chondrosarcoma, invasive meningioma, or metastases. One clue to look for is the presence of vascular pulsation artifacts propagating from the aneurysm along the phase-encoding direction. Care must be taken to prevent inadvertent biopsies or resections of these aneurysms. CT angiography, MR angiography, or conventional angiogram should also be obtained to confirm the diagnosis, evaluate the aneurysm neck, and assess the context of the aneurysm with regards to the parent vessel and adjacent neurovascular structures for endovascular or surgical planning (**Fig. 18**).

If left untreated, these aneurysm are associated with a high rate of thromboembolic events, seen in up to 50% of patients.[123] Because the petrous ICA aneurysms are often completely enclosed by bone, surgical access for ligation is difficult and endovascular therapy is the preferred approach.[123,124,126] This is performed with a variety of techniques, such as flow-diverting stent placement, coil embolization, or progressive flow reduction.

SUMMARY

The skull base features complex anatomy, containing many different tissue types, foramina, canals, and synchondroses, predisposing it to a variety of anatomic variants and masses, benign and malignant. Skull base lesions can demonstrate a variety of confusing appearances on imaging, creating diagnostic dilemmas. It is important to be familiar with imaging appearances of common mimickers of malignant neoplasm in the skull base to be able to accurately diagnose them and prevent unnecessary imaging follow-up, biopsies, or interventions.

CLINICS CARE POINTS

- Familiarity with the common normal variant and benign lesions occurring in the skull base may prevent confusion with more sinister pathologies, reducing healthcare waste and patient stress.

- Anatomic variants in the skull base are common, occurring along the course of the notochord and craniopharyngeal canal.

- Ill-defined hypointensity on T2 with surrounding inflammatory changes can suggest skull base osteomyelitis or chronic inflammatory process.

- Petrous internal carotid artery aneurysm is a "must not miss" diagnosis with varied imaging appearances on MRI depending on the flow and amount of thrombus formation.

- Other benign mimics in the skull base have characteristic appearances, including arrested pneumatization of the sphenoid sinus, cephalocele, fibrous dysplasia, ecchordosis physaliphora, and invasive pituitary adenoma.

DISCLOSURES

The authors have nothing to disclose.

REFERENCES

1. Raut A, Naphade P, Chawla A. Imaging of skull base: pictorial essay. Indian J Radiol Imaging 2012;22:305.

2. Borges A. Imaging of the central skull base. Neuro-imaging Clin N Am 2009;19:441–68.

3. Thust SC, Yousry T. Imaging of skull base tumours. Rep Pract Oncol Radiother 2016;21:304–18.

4. Kunimatsu A, Kunimatsu N. Skull base tumors and tumor-like lesions: a pictorial review. Pol J Radiol 2017;82:398–409.

5. Currarino G. Canalis basilaris medianus and related defects of the basiocciput. AJNR Am J Neuroradiol 1988;9:208–11.

6. Jacquemin C, Bosley TM, al Saleh M, et al. Canalis basilaris medianus: MRI. Neuroradiology 2000;42:121–3.

7. Hughes ML, Carty AT, White FE. Persistent hypophyseal (craniopharyngeal) canal. Br J Radiol 1999;72:204–6.

8. Abele TA, Salzman KL, Harnsberger HR, et al. Craniopharyngeal canal and its spectrum of pathology. Am J Neuroradiol 2014;35:772–7.

9. Zhang WH, Yen WC. A new bony canal on the clival surface of the occipital bone. Acta Anat (Basel) 1987;128:63–6.

10. Syed AZ, Zahedpasha S, Rathore SA, et al. Evaluation of canalis basilaris medianus using cone-beam computed tomography. Imaging Sci Dent 2016;46:141–4.

11. Bayrak S, Göller Bulut D, Orhan K. Prevalence of anatomical variants in the clivus: fossa navicularis magna, canalis basilaris medianus, and craniopharyngeal canal. Surg Radiol Anat 2019;41:477–83.

12. Madeline LA, Elster AD. Postnatal development of the central skull base: normal variants. Radiology 1995;196:757–63.

13. Paraskevas GK, Tsitsopoulos PP, Ioannidis OM. Incidence and purpose of the clival canal, a "neglected" skull base canal. Acta Neurochir (Wien) 2013;155:139–40.

14. Tubbs RS, Griessenauer CJ, Loukas M, et al. The enigmatic clival canal: anatomy and clinical significance. Childs Nerv Syst 2010;26:1207–10.

15. Jalšovec D, Vinter I. Clinical significance of a bony canal of the clivus. Eur Arch Otorhinolaryngol 1999; 256:160–1.

16. Nguyen RP, Salzman KL, Stambuk HE, et al. Extra-osseous chordoma of the nasopharynx. Am J Neuroradiol 2009;30:803–7.

17. Martinez CR, Hemphill JM, Hodges FJ, et al. Basioccipital meningocele. AJNR Am J Neuroradiol 1981;2:100–2.

18. Hemphill M, Freeman JM, Martinez CR, et al. A new, treatable source of recurrent meningitis: basioccipital meningocele. Pediatrics 1982;70:941–3.

19. Morabito R, Longo M, Rossi A, et al. Pharyngeal enterogenous cyst associated with canalis basilaris medianus in a newborn. Pediatr Radiol 2013; 43:512–5.

20. Lohman BD, Sarikaya B, McKinney AM, et al. Not the typical Tornwaldt's cyst this time? A nasopharyngeal cyst associated with canalis basilaris medianus. Br J Radiol 2011;84:e169–71.

21. Khairy S, Almubarak AO, Aloraidi A, et al. Canalis basalis medianus with cerebrospinal fluid leak: rare presentation and literature review. Br J Neurosurg 2019;33:432–3.

22. Ko AL, Gabikian P, Perkins JA, et al. Endoscopic repair of a rare basioccipital meningocele associated with recurrent meningitis: case report. J Neurosurg Pediatr 2010;6:188–92.

23. Syed AZ, Mupparapu M. Fossa navicularis magna detection on cone-beam computed tomography. Imaging Sci Dent 2016;46(1):47–51.

24. Beltramello A, Puppini G, El-Dalati G, et al. Fossa navicularis magna. AJNR Am J Neuroradiol 1998;19: 1796–8.

25. Ray B, Kalthur S, Kumar B, et al. Morphological variations in the basioccipital region of the South Indian skull. Nepal J Med Sci 2015;3:124–8.

26. Cankal F, Ugur HC, Tekdemir I, et al. Fossa navicularis: anatomic variation at the skull base. Clin Anat 2004;17:118–22.

27. Ersan N. Prevalence and morphometric features of fossa navicularis on cone beam computed tomography in Turkish population. Folia Morphol 2017;76:6.

28. Ginat DT, Ellika SK, Corrigan J. Multidetector-row computed tomography imaging of variant skull base foramina. J Comput Assist Tomogr 2013;37:5.

29. Prabhu SP, Zinkus T, Cheng AG, et al. Clival osteomyelitis resulting from spread of infection through the fossa navicularis magna in a child. Pediatr Radiol 2009;39:995–8.

30. Alalade AF, Briganti G, Mckenzie J-L, et al. Fossa navicularis in a pediatric patient: anatomical skull base variant with clinical implications. J Neurosurg Pediatr 2018;22:523–7.

31. Segal N, Atamne E, Shelef I, et al. Intracranial infection caused by spreading through the fossa naviclaris magna: a case report and review of the literature. Int J Pediatr Otorhinolaryngol 2013;77:1919–21.

32. Currarino G, Maravilla KR, Salyer KE. Transsphenoidal canal (large craniopharyngeal canal) and its pathologic implications. AJNR Am J Neuroradiol 1985;6:39–43.

33. Arey LB. The craniopharyngeal canal reviewed and reinterpreted. Anat Rec 1950;106:1–16.

34. Larsen JL, Bassøe HH. Transsphenoidal meningocele with hypothalamic insufficiency. Neuroradiology 1979;18:205–9.

35. Hori A, Schmidt D, Rickels E. Pharyngeal pituitary: development, malformation, and tumorigenesis. Acta Neuropathol 1999;98:262–72.

36. Hooper AC. Sphenoidal defects: a possible cause of cerebrospinal fluid rhinorrhoea. J Neurol Neurosurg Psychiatry 1971;34:739–42.

37. Rajasekar G, Nair P, Abraham M, et al. Endoscopic endonasal repair of a persistent craniopharyngeal

canal and sphenoid meningoencephalocele: case report and review of literature. World Neurosurg 2019;122:196–202.

38. Lingappa L, Konanki R, Varma R, et al. Persistent craniopharyngeal canal: a rare cause for recurrent meningitis in pediatric population. Ann Indian Acad Neurol 2019;0:0.

39. Habermann S, Silva AHD, Aquilina K, et al. A persistent craniopharyngeal canal with recurrent bacterial meningitis: case report and literature review. Childs Nerv Syst 2021;37:699–702.

40. Poonia SK, Cazzador D, Kaufman AC, et al. Disorders involving a persistent craniopharyngeal canal: a case series. J Neurol Surg B Skull Base 2020;81: 562–6.

41. Kaushik C, Ramakrishnaiah R, Angtuaco EJ. Ectopic pituitary adenoma in persistent craniopharyngeal canal: case report and literature review. J Comput Assist Tomogr 2010;34:612–4.

42. Ekinci G, Kiliç T, Baltacioğlu F, et al. Transsphenoidal (large craniopharyngeal) canal associated with a normally functioning pituitary gland and nasopharyngeal extension, hyperprolactinemia, and hypothalamic hamartoma. Am J Roentgenol 2003;180:76–7.

43. Kumar S, Pujari VS, Munshi M, et al. Neonatal respiratory distress produced by a nasopharyngeal glioma with a persistent craniopharyngeal canal. J Med Imaging Radiat Oncol 2020;64:824–6.

44. Chen CJ. Suprasellar and infrasellar craniopharyngioma with a persistent craniopharyngeal canal: case report and review of the literature. Neuroradiology 2001;43:760–2.

45. Welker KM, DeLone DR, Lane JI, et al. Arrested pneumatization of the skull base: imaging characteristics. Am J Roentgenol 2008;190:1691–6.

46. Scuderi AJ, Harnsberger HR, Boyer RS. Pneumatization of the paranasal sinuses: normal features of importance to the accurate interpretation of CT scans and MR images. Am J Roentgenol 1993; 160:1101–4.

47. Spaeth J, Krügelstein U, Schlöndorff G. The paranasal sinuses in CT-imaging: development from birth to age 25. Int J Pediatr Otorhinolaryngol 1997;39:25–40.

48. Yonetsu K, Watanabe M, Nakamura T. Age-related expansion and reduction in aeration of the sphenoid sinus: volume assessment by helical CT scanning. AJNR Am J Neuroradiol 2000;21(1):179–82. [Epub ahead of print].

49. Shah RK, Dhingra JK, Carter BL, et al. Paranasal sinus development: a radiographic study. Laryngoscope 2003;113:205–9.

50. Jalali E, Tadinada A. Arrested pneumatization of the sphenoid sinus mimicking intraosseous lesions of the skull base. Imaging Sci Dent 2015;45:67–72.

51. Arpaci T. Arrested pneumatization of the sphenoid sinus mimicking skull base tumours: MRI

prevalence in children with haematologic diseases. Int J Neurosci 2018;128:1040–3.

52. Tuncay OC, Ho D, Barker MK. Oxygen tension regulates osteoblast function. Am J Orthod Dentofacial Orthop 1994;105:457–63.

53. Nager GT. Cephaloceles. Laryngoscope 1987;97: 77–84.

54. Simpson DA, David DJ, White J. Cephaloceles: treatment, outcome, and antenatal diagnosis. Neurosurgery 1984;15:14–21.

55. Baradaran N, Nejat F, Baradaran N, et al. Cephalocele: report of 55 cases over 8 years. Pediatr Neurosurg 2009;45:461–6.

56. Lo BWY, Kulkarni AV, Rutka JT, et al. Clinical predictors of developmental outcome in patients with cephaloceles: clinical article. J Neurosurg Pediatr 2008;2:254–7.

57. Martínez-Lage JF, Poza M, Sola J, et al. The child with a cephalocele: etiology, neuroimaging, and outcome. Childs Nerv Syst 1996;12(9):540–50.

58. Budorick NE, Pretorius DH, McGahan JP, et al. Cephalocele detection in utero: sonographic and clinical features. Ultrasound Obstet Gynecol 1995;5:77–85.

59. Brown MS, Sheridan-Pereira M. Outlook for the child with a cephalocele. Pediatrics 1992;90:914–9.

60. Wininger SJ, Donnenfeld AE. Syndromes identified in fetuses with prenatally diagnosed cephaloceles. Prenat Diagn 1994;14:839–43.

61. Alkhaibary A, Musawnaq F, Almuntashri M, et al. Bilateral petrous apex cephaloceles: is surgical intervention indicated? Int J Surg Case Rep 2020; 72:373–6.

62. Deasy NP, Jarosz JM, Sarraj SA, et al. Intrasphenoid cephalocele: MRI in two cases. Neuroradiology 1999;41:497–500.

63. Alonso RC, de la Peña MJ, Caicoya AG, et al. Spontaneous skull base meningoencephaloceles and cerebrospinal fluid fistulas. RadioGraphics 2013;33:553–70.

64. Lustig LR, Holliday MJ, McCarthy EF, et al. Fibrous dysplasia involving the skull base and temporal bone. Arch Otolaryngol Neck Surg 2001;127: 1239.

65. Schreiber A, Villaret AB, Maroldi R, et al. Fibrous dysplasia of the sinonasal tract and adjacent skull base. Curr Opin Otolaryngol Head Neck Surg 2012;20:45–52.

66. Fitzpatrick KA, Taljanovic MS, Speer DP, et al. Imaging findings of fibrous dysplasia with histopathologic and intraoperative correlation. Am J Roentgenol 2004;182:1389–98.

67. Amit M, Fliss DM, Gil Z. Fibrous dysplasia of the sphenoid and skull base. Otolaryngol Clin North Am 2011;44:891–902.

68. Kushchayeva YS, Kushchayev SV, Glushko TY, et al. Fibrous dysplasia for radiologists: beyond

ground glass bone matrix. Insights Imaging 2018; 9:1035–56.

69. Brown EW, Megerian CA, McKenna MJ, et al. Fibrous dysplasia of the temporal bone: imaging findings. Am J Roentgenol 1995;164:679–82.

70. Chong VFH, Khoo JBK, Fan Y-F. Fibrous dysplasia involving the base of the skull. Am J Roentgenol 2002;178:717–20.

71. Windeyer BW. Chordoma. Proc R Soc Med 1959; 52:1088–100.

72. Mehnert F, Beschorner R, Kuker W, et al. Retroclival ecchordosis physaliphora: MR imaging and review of the literature. AJNR Am J Neuroradiol 2004; 25(10):1851–5. [Epub ahead of print].

73. Watanabe A, Yanagita M, Ishii R, et al. Magnetic resonance imaging of ecchordosis physaliphora–case report. Neurol Med Chir (Tokyo) 1994;34: 448–50.

74. Park HH, Lee K-S, Ahn SJ, et al. Ecchordosis physaliphora: typical and atypical radiologic features. Neurosurg Rev 2017;40:87–94.

75. Adamek D, Malec M, Grabska N, et al. Ecchordosis physaliphora: a case report and a review of notochord-derived lesions. Neurol Neurochir Pol 2011;45:169–73.

76. Macdonald RL, Cusimano MD, Deck JH, et al. Cerebrospinal fluid fistula secondary to ecchordosis physaliphora. Neurosurgery 1990;26:515–8 [discussion: 518-519].

77. Lagman C, Varshneya K, Sarmiento JM, et al. Proposed diagnostic criteria, classification schema, and review of literature of notochord-derived ecchordosis physaliphora. Cureus 2016. https://doi. org/10.7759/cureus.547.

78. Takeyama J, Hayashi T, Shirane R. Notochordal remnant-derived mass: ecchordosis physaliphora or chordoma? Pathology (Phila) 2006;38:599–600.

79. Derakhshani A, Livingston S, William C, et al. Spontaneous, intrasphenoidal rupture of ecchordosis physaliphora with pneumocephalus captured during serial imaging and clinical follow-up: pathoanatomic features and management. World Neurosurg 2020;141:85–90.

80. Ng S-H, Ko S-F, Wan Y-L, et al. Cervical ecchordosis physaliphora: CT and MR features. Br J Radiol 1998;71(843):329–31. [Epub ahead of print].

81. Ghimire P, Shapey J, Bodi I, et al. Spontaneous tension pneumocephalus and pneumoventricle in ecchordosis physaliphora: case report of a rare presentation and review of the literature. Br J Neurosurg 2020;34:537–42.

82. Sun R, Ajam Y, Campbell G, et al. A rare case of ecchordosis physaliphora presenting with headache, abducens nerve palsy, and intracranial hypertension. Cureus 2020. https://doi.org/10.7759/ cureus.8843.

83. Toda H, Kondo A, Iwasaki K. Neuroradiological characteristics of ecchordosis physaliphora: case report and review of the literature. J Neurosurg 1998;89:830–4.

84. Georgalas C, Terzakis D, Tsikna M, et al. Ecchordosis physaliphora: a cautionary tale. J Laryngol Otol 2020;134:46–51.

85. Kurokawa H, Miura S, Goto T. Ecchordosis physaliphora arising from the cervical vertebra, the CT and MRI appearance. Neuroradiology 1988;30:81–3.

86. Alkan O, Yildirim T, Kizilkiliç O, et al. A case of ecchordosis physaliphora presenting with an intratumoral hemorrhage. Turk Neurosurg 2009;19:293–6.

87. Appel JG, Bergsneider M, Vinters H, et al. Acromegaly due to an ectopic pituitary adenoma in the clivus: case report and review of literature. Pituitary 2012;15:53–6.

88. Wong K, Raisanen J, Taylor SL, et al. Pituitary adenoma as an unsuspected clival tumor. Am J Surg Pathol 1995;19:900–3.

89. Sarkar S, Chacko AG, Chacko G. Clinicopathological correlates of extrasellar growth patterns in pituitary adenomas. J Clin Neurosci 2015;22:1173–7.

90. Hagiwara A, Inoue Y, Wakasa K, et al. Comparison of growth hormone–producing and non–growth hormone–producing pituitary adenomas: imaging characteristics and pathologic correlation. Radiology 2003;228:533–8.

91. Zada G, Lin N, Laws ER. Patterns of extrasellar extension in growth hormone–secreting and nonfunctional pituitary macroadenomas. Neurosurg Focus 2010;29:E4.

92. Edal AL, Skjödt K, Nepper-Rasmussen HJ. SIPAP–a new MR classification for pituitary adenomas. Suprasellar, infrasellar, parasellar, anterior and posterior. Acta Radiol 1997;38:30–6.

93. Gao A, Bai J, Cheng J, et al. Differentiating skull base chordomas and invasive pituitary adenomas with conventional MRI. Acta Radiol 2018;59:1358–64.

94. Kuo AH, Nuñez DB. Giant pituitary adenoma with inferior petrosal sinus, jugular foramen, and hypoglossal canal extension. JAMA Otolaryngol Neck Surg 2020;146:82.

95. Riccio L, Donofrio CA, Tomacelli G, et al. Ectopic GH-secreting pituitary adenoma of the clivus: systematic literature review of a challenging tumour. Pituitary 2020;23:457–66.

96. Mudd PA, Hohensee S, Lillehei KO, et al. Ectopic pituitary adenoma of the clivus presenting with apoplexy: case report and review of the literature. Clin Neuropathol 2012;31:24–30.

97. Abele TA, Yetkin ZF, Raisanen JM, et al. Non-pituitary origin sellar tumours mimicking pituitary macroadenomas. Clin Radiol 2012;67:821–7.

98. Donovan JL, Nesbit GM. Distinction of masses involving the sella and suprasellar space:

specificity of imaging features. Am J Roentgenol 1996;167:597–603.

99. Anand P, Chwalisz BK. Inflammatory disorders of the skull base: a review. Curr Neurol Neurosci Rep 2019;19:96.

100. Khan M, Quadri SQ, Kazmi A, et al. A comprehensive review of skull base osteomyelitis: diagnostic and therapeutic challenges among various presentations. Asian J Neurosurg 2018;13:959.

101. Álvarez Jáñez F, Barriga LQ, Iñigo TR, et al. Diagnosis of skull base osteomyelitis. RadioGraphics 2021;41:156–74.

102. Jain N, Jasper A, Vanjare HA, et al. The role of imaging in skull base osteomyelitis: reviewed. Clin Imaging 2020;67:62–7.

103. Sokołowski J, Lachowska M, Karchier E, et al. Skull base osteomyelitis: factors implicating clinical outcome. Acta Neurol Belg 2019;119:431–7.

104. Ozgen B, Oguz KK, Cila A. Diffusion MR imaging features of skull base osteomyelitis compared with skull base malignancy. Am J Neuroradiol 2011;32:179–84.

105. Ryu G, Cho H-J, Lee KE, et al. Clinical significance of IgG4 in sinonasal and skull base inflammatory pseudotumor. Eur Arch Otorhinolaryngol 2019;276:2465–73.

106. Alyono JC, Shi Y, Berry GJ, et al. Inflammatory pseudotumors of the skull base: meta-analysis. Otol Neurotol 2015;36(8):1432–8.

107. Marinelli JP, Marvisi C, Vaglio A, et al. Manifestations of skull base IgG4-related disease: a multi-institutional study. Laryngoscope 2020;130:2574–80.

108. Cain RB, Colby TV, Balan V, et al. Perplexing lesions of the sinonasal cavity and skull base: IgG4-related and similar inflammatory diseases. Otolaryngol Neck Surg 2014;151:496–502.

109. Han MH, Chi JG, Kim MS, et al. Fibrosing inflammatory pseudotumors involving the skull base: MR and CT manifestations with histopathologic comparison. AJNR Am J Neuroradiol 1996;17(3):515–21. [Epub ahead of print].

110. Desai SV, Spinazzi EF, Fang CH, et al. Sinonasal and ventral skull base Inflammatory pseudotumor: a systematic review: skull base inflammatory pseudotumor. Laryngoscope 2015;125:813–21.

111. Kiessling PT, Marinelli JP, Peters PA, et al. Cranial base manifestations of granulomatosis with polyangiitis. Otolaryngol Neck Surg 2020;162:666–73.

112. Keni SP, Wiley EL, Dutra JC, et al. Skull base Wegener's granulomatosis resulting in multiple cranial neuropathies. Am J Otolaryngol 2005;26:146–9.

113. Sharma A, Deshmukh S, Shaikh A, et al. Wegener's granulomatosis mimicking skull base osteomyelitis. J Laryngol Otol 2012;126:203–6.

114. Todd Andrews J, Kountakis SE. Wegener's granulomatosis of the skull base. Am J Otolaryngol 1996;17:349–52.

115. Moore KR, Fischbein NJ, Harnsberger HR, et al. Petrous apex cephaloceles. AJNR Am J Neuroradiol 2001;22(10):1867–71. [Epub ahead of print].

116. Connor SEJ, Leung R, Natas S. Imaging of the petrous apex: a pictorial review. Br J Radiol 2008;81:427–35.

117. Jamjoom DZ, Alorainy IA. The association between petrous apex cephalocele and empty sella. Surg Radiol Anat 2015;37:1179–82.

118. Schmalfuss IM, Camp M. Skull base: pseudolesion or true lesion? Eur Radiol 2008;18:1232–43.

119. Moore KR, Harnsberger HR, Shelton C, et al. Leave me alone lesions of the petrous apex. AJNR Am J Neuroradiol 1998;19(4):733–8. [Epub ahead of print].

120. Roland PS, Meyerhoff WL, Judge LO, et al. Asymmetric pneumatization of the petrous apex. Otolaryngol Neck Surg 1990;103:80–8.

121. Arriaga MA. Petrous apex effusion: a clinical disorder. Laryngoscope 2006;116:1349 56.

122. Yildirim M, Senturk S, Guzel E, et al. Bilateral symptomatic petrous apex effusion. Indian J Otolaryngol Head Neck Surg 2010;62:186–8.

123. Chapman PR, Gaddamanugu S, Bag AK, et al. Vascular lesions of the central skull base region. Semin Ultrasound CT MRI 2013;34:459–75.

124. Moonis G, Hwang CJ, Ahmed T, et al. Otologic manifestations of petrous carotid aneurysms. AJNR Am J Neuroradiol 2005;26(6):1324–7. [Epub ahead of print].

125. Tamada T, Mikami T, Akiyama Y, et al. Giant petrous internal carotid aneurysm causing epistaxis: a case report. J Clin Neurosci 2018;58:221–3.

126. Borha A, Patron V, Huet H, et al. Endovascular management of a giant petrous internal carotid artery aneurysm in a child. Case report and literature review. Childs Nerv Syst 2019;35:183–6.

127. Liu JK, Gottfried ON, Amini A, et al. Aneurysms of the petrous internal carotid artery: anatomy, origins, and treatment. Neurosurg Focus 2004;17:1–9.

128. Murai Y, Shirokane K, Kitamura T, et al. Petrous internal carotid artery aneurysm: a systematic review. J Nippon Med Sch 2020;87:172–83.

129. Kim S-M, Kim C-H, Lee C-Y. Petrous carotid aneurysm causing pulsatile tinnitus: case report and review of the literature. J Cerebrovasc Endovasc Neurosurg 2018;20:35–9.

130. Cano-Duran AJ, Sanchez Reyes JM, Corbalan Sevilla MT, et al. Carotid petrous segment aneurysm presenting as hypoglossal nerve palsy. Neuroradiology 2021;63:447–50.

131. Hamamoto Filho PT, Machado VC, Macedo-de-Freitas CC. A giant aneurysm from the petrous carotid presenting with isolated peripheral facial palsy. Rev Assoc Médica Bras 2013;59:531–3.

Normal Anatomic Structures, Variants, and Mimics of the Temporal Bone

Gul Moonis, MD[a,*], Daniel T. Ginat, MD, MS[b]

KEYWORDS

- Temporal bone • Mimics • Cochlear cleft • Otosclerosis • Pseudofractures

KEY POINTS

- There are numerous sutures and fissures in the temporal bone, which should not be mistaken for fractures.
- Not all mastoid air cell opacification represents mastoiditis.
- Look for sigmoid sinus bony dehiscence and pseudotumor cerebri as potential causes of pulsatile tinnitus.
- Besides ossicular lesions, compromise of the round window and otospongiosis can lead to conductive hearing loss.

TEMPORAL BONE FRACTURE MIMICS

Temporal bone pseudofractures can be categorized as intrinsic fissures, extrinsic fissures, and intrinsic channels[1,2] (Table 1). There are 4 intrinsic fissures surrounding the external auditory canal. These include the tympanosquamous, petrotympanic, and petrosquamous fissures (Fig. 1) in addition to the tympanomastoid suture. The extrinsic fissures refer to the sutures that separate the temporal bone from the surrounding calvarium. These include the occipitomastoid, petrooccipital, sphenosquamosal, and sphenopetrosal sutures (Fig. 2). In general, sutures can be differentiated from true fractures by virtue of their corticated margins and zigzag course (see Fig. 2). The intrinsic channels include the petromastoid canal, hiatus of the facial canal, singular canal, vestibular aqueduct, cochlear aqueduct, inferior tympanic canaliculus, and mastoid canaliculus (Fig. 3).

LUCENCY IN THE OTIC CAPSULE

Otosclerosis is an osteodystrophy of the otic capsule, which is usually bilateral and affects females more than males. Histopathologically, the normally dense middle layer of endochondral bone is replaced by spongy vascular bone. This is responsible for the classic lucent appearance of otosclerosis lesions in the otic capsule. Over time, the spongy bone can become more sclerotic. The most common location for otosclerosis is a small cleft just anterior to the oval window known as the fissula antefenestrum (fenestral otosclerosis). When the abnormality extends to the remainder of the bony labyrinth, this is termed retrofenestral otosclerosis. On computed tomography (CT) scan, lucency anterior to the oval window at the fissula antefenestrum and a halo of lucency surrounding the cochlea are characteristically seen in fenestral and retrofenestral otosclerosis, respectively (Fig. 4C, D).

The cochlear cleft is a transient developmental finding on temporal bone CT in younger children related to incomplete endochondral ossification of the otic capsule, which progresses independently of membranous and bony labyrinth development.[3,4] While apparent in 80% of infants younger than 1 year of age, it becomes less conspicuous with age. The cochlear cleft appears as

a Department of Radiology, NYU Langone Medical Center, 222 East 41st Street, 5th Floor, New York, NY 10017, USA; b Department of Radiology, University of Chicago, 5841 S Maryland Avenue, Chicago, IL 60637, USA
* Corresponding author.
E-mail address: gul.moonis@nyulangone.org

Neuroimag Clin N Am 32 (2022) 345–361
https://doi.org/10.1016/j.nic.2022.01.007
1052-5149/22/© 2022 Elsevier Inc. All rights reserved.

Table 1
Temporal pseudo fracture descriptions

	Structure	Description
Intrinsic fissures	Tympanosquamous	Separates the tympanic bone from the squamous bone and is continuous medially with the petrotympanic and petrosquamous fissures
	Petrotympanic	Extends from the temporomandibular joint to the tympanic cavity and transmits the chorda tympani
	Petrosquamous	Best seen on coronal reformats as a small gap in the tegmen tympani
	Tympanomastoid suture	Cleft posterior to the external auditory canal; it separates the external auditory canal from the mastoid
Extrinsic fissures	Occipitomastoid	Posterior to the mastoid; separates from the occipital bone
	Petrooccipital	Extends from the petrous apex to the pars nervosa of the jugular foramen
	Sphenosquamosal	Located lateral to the foramen spinosum, between the greater wing of the sphenoid bone and the squamous portion of the temporal bone
	Sphenopetrosal	The sphenopetrosal suture is located posterior to the foramen ovale between the greater wing of the sphenoid and the petrous apex
Intrinsic channels	Petromastoid (subarcuate) canal	Narrow passage between the limbs of the superior semicircular canal that connects the mastoid antrum with the posterior cranial fossa and contains the subarcuate blood vessels and extension of the dura
	Hiatus of the facial canal	Located on the anterior surface of the petrous bone, contiguous to the geniculate ganglion, and transmits the greater petrosal nerve
	Singular canal	Extends from the posterior wall of the internal auditory canal to the ampulla of the posterior semicircular canal and contains the singular nerve, which is a branch of the inferior vestibular nerve
	Vestibular aqueduct	Extends from the medial aspect of the posterior wall of the vestibule to the dura along the posterior aspect of the petrous apex and contains a small vein and a projection of the membranous labyrinth
	Cochlear aqueduct	Funnel-shaped perilymphatic duct that extends from the subarachnoid space to the basal turn of the cochlea
	Inferior tympanic canaliculus	Channel for the inferior tympanic branch of the glossopharyngeal nerve from the pars nervosa into the middle ear
	Mastoid canaliculus	Located just above the stylomastoid foramen, where it allows the passage of the auricular branch of the vagus nerve from the pars vascularis to the facial canal

a lucent crescentic area within the middle of the otic capsule parallel to the basal turn of the cochlea, underneath the cochleariform process, and is typically bilateral (**Fig. 4**A, B). It should be noted that although this structure may vary in size, its form is constant. Although incomplete endochondral ossification of the cochlear cleft can resemble otosclerosis, it lacks associated clinical and audiologic manifestations.

Osteogenesis imperfecta is a rare inherited disorder of connective tissues caused by an error in collagen type 1 formation. On CT scan, lucency in the pericochlear otic capsule may be seen and can mimic the findings of otosclerosis (see **Fig. 4**E, F). The disease can progress to involve the facial nerve canal. These patients have characteristic clinical features including blue sclera and ligamentous laxity. Histopathologically, there is

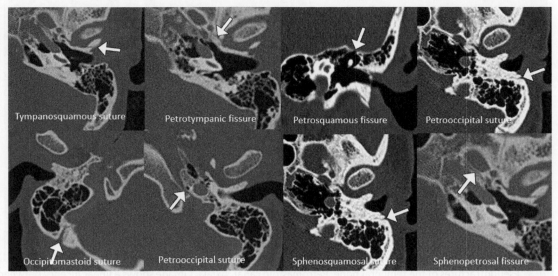

Fig. 1. Pseudofractures of the temporal Bone. Tympanosquamous suture. The axial CT image shows a linear lucency anterior to the left external auditory canal (*arrow*). Petrotympanic fissure. Axial CT image shows a lucency that extends from the temporomandibular joint to the tympanic cavity (*arrow*). Petrosquamous fissure. Coronal CT image shows a small gap in the tegmen tympani (*arrow*). Tympanomastoid fissure. Axial CT image shows a cleft posterior to the external auditory canal (*arrow*). Occipitomastoid suture. Axial CT image shows a gap between the mastoid and the occipital bone (*arrow*). Petrooccipital suture. Axial CT image shows a gap between the petrous bone and clivus, toward the jugular foramen (*arrow*). Sphenosquamosal suture. Axial CT image shows a linear lucency lateral to the foramen spinosum between the greater wing of the sphenoid bone and the squamous portion of the temporal bone (*arrow*). Sphenopetrosal fissure. Axial CT image shows a gap between the foramen ovale between the greater wing of the sphenoid and the carotid canal (*arrow*).

presence of thickened and undermineralized bone.

Other differential diagnoses for this lucent appearance of the otic capsule include Paget disease and otosyphilis.[5]

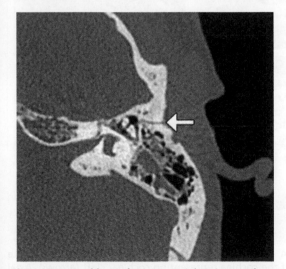

Fig. 2. Temporal bone fracture. Axial CT image shows a fracture that traverses the left mastoid bone (*arrow*) and incudo-malleal separation.

Overuse of the Term Mastoiditis in Radiology Reports

Mastoiditis is a clinical entity that represents infection of the middle ear spreading to the mastoid air cells. Complicated acute mastoiditis or coalescent acute mastoiditis is characterized by disease spreading from the mucosa into the bone and is an otological emergency. Clinically this is evidenced by postauricular tenderness, erythema, and protrusion of the auricle. CT imaging demonstrates mastoid septal and cortical erosion, subperiosteal abscess, and intracranial abscesses (Fig. 5A). On MRI, complicated acute mastoiditis is seen as mastoid T2 hyperintensity with enhancement and restricted diffusion (intramastoid empyema) (Fig. 6). Isolated mastoid opacification/effusion without osseous destruction or abscess formation (Fig. 5B) is uncommon in the setting of complicated mastoiditis, but is seen commonly in patients with uncomplicated acute otitis externa and media. Moreover, incidental mastoid opacification in asymptomatic and intubated individuals is also seen. Chronic mastoid inflammation usually manifests as mastoid opacification with sclerosis (Fig. 5C).

Mastoid opacification without bony destruction even in asymptomatic individuals is often referred

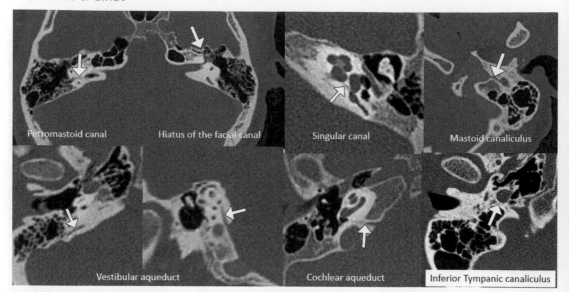

Fig. 3. Pseudofractures of the temporal bone. Petromastoid canal. Axial CT image shows a linear lucency between the 2 limbs of the superior semicircular canal (*arrow*). Hiatus of the facial canal. Axial CT image shows a linear gap for the greater petrosal nerve (*arrow*) in the petrous bone anterior to the geniculate ganglion singular canal. Axial CT image shows a lucency that extends from the posterior aspect of the internal auditory canal to the ampulla of the posterior semicircular canal (*arrow*). Vestibular aqueduct. Axial (*A*) and Poschl (*B*) CT images show a vertical cleft in the posterior petrous bone (*arrows*). Cochlear aqueduct. Axial CT image shows a fine linear lucency that extends from the basal turn of the cochlea, adjacent to the round window, and slightly widens medially toward the subarachnoid space (*arrow*). Inferior tympanic canaliculus. Axial CT image shows a fine linear lucency situated between the carotid canal and the jugular foramen (*arrow*). Mastoid canaliculus. Axial CT image shows a fine lucency located medial to the mastoid segment of the facial nerve canal, just above the stylomastoid foramen (*arrow*).

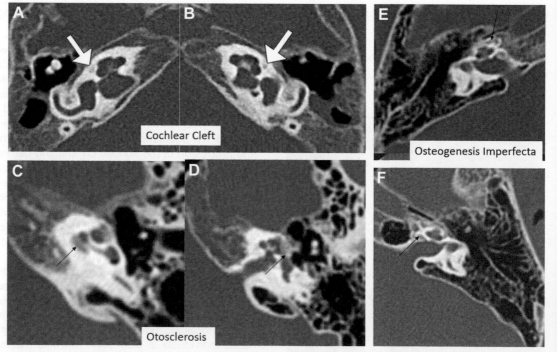

Fig. 4. Otic capsule lucency. Bilateral axial CT images (*A, B*) obtained in a 5-month-old infant show punctate lucency in the otic capsules lateral to the middle turns of the cochlea representing cochlear cleft (*arrows*). Axial CT images (*C, D*) show lucency at the fissula ante fenestram (*arrow D*) and in the pericochlear region (*arrow C*) representing fenestral and retrofenestral otosclerosis respectively. Axial CT scan in a patient with osteogenesis imperfecta type I (*E, F*) demonstrate bilateral lucency surrounding the peri-cochlear otic capsule (*arrow*), which mimics retrofenestral otosclerosis.

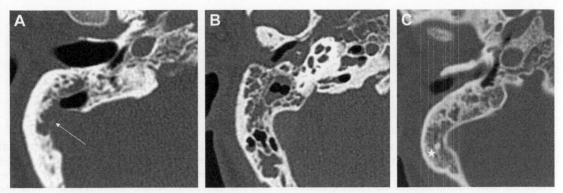

Fig. 5. Different causes of mastoid opacification. Axial CT scan in a patient with coalescent mastoiditis (A) reveals erosion of the mastoid septations and the inner cortex of the mastoid (arrow). The patient presented acutely with ear pain and discharge. Axial CT in patient with uncomplicated otomastoiditis from acute otitis media demonstrates fluid in the mastoid air cells (B) and middle ear with a fluid level. Note preservation of septations and the inner and outer mastoid cortex. Axial CT scan in a patient with chronic otomastoiditis (C) shows sclerosis (*) and opacification of the mastoid air cells on the right.

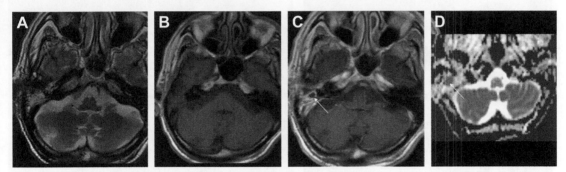

Fig. 6. Coalescent mastoiditis on MRI. Axial T2-weighted (A), and pre- (B) and postcontrast (C) T1-weighted images demonstrate T2 hyperintense signal in the right mastoid air cells with corresponding enhancement in a patient who presented with acute ear pain, erythema, and fever. There is a focus of nonenhancement in the anterior mastoid air cells (arrow in C), which corresponds to restricted diffusion on the ADC map (arrow D), which represents an intramastoid empyema. Note that in a patient with a different more chronic clinical picture, the focus of restricted diffusion could also represent cholesteatoma.

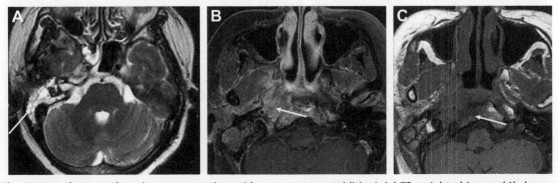

Fig. 7. Nasopharyngeal carcinoma presenting with serous otomastoiditis. Axial T2-weighted image (A) demonstrates fluid signal in the right mastoid air cells and middle ear cavity. On the pre- and postcontrast images, the obstructive mass in the right nasopharynx fossa of Rosenmuller is demonstrated (arrow in B). On the precontrast T1-weighted image (C), extension into the clivus is nicely demonstrated as replacement of normal fatty marrow by abnormal signal. Right carotid encasement is also seen.

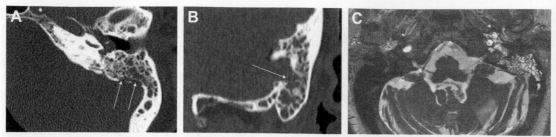

Fig. 8. CSF leak from prominent arachnoid granulation in the posterior petrous ridge. Axial and coronal CT (*A*, *B*) imaging demonstrates prominent arachnoid granulations along the left posterior petrous ridge with opacified mastoid air cells and middle ear. Axial 3D-FIESTA image (*C*) demonstrates left otomastoid fluid signal. This represented CSF leak from erosion of arachnoid granulations into the mastoid air cells. One needs to scrutinize the study for other signs of idiopathic intracranial hypertension.

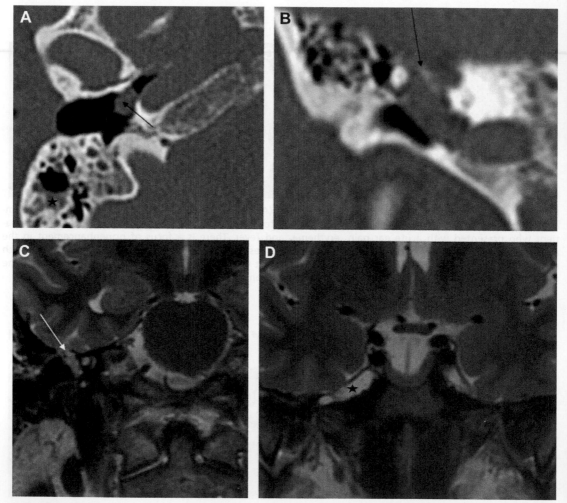

Fig. 9. Meningocele presenting as a pulsatile red mass on otoscopy. Axial and coronal CT images (*A*, *B*) demonstrate lobulated soft tissue density in the right middle ear cleft with erosion of the tegmen tympani (*arrow* in B). MRI confirms the presence of a meningoencephalocele on the coronal T2-weighted image (*arrow* in C). Signs of increased intracranial hypertension are also noted on another coronal T2-weighted image (*D*) with prominent Meckel cave on the right (*) and partially empty sella.

to as mastoiditis by radiologists in their reports. However, to the primary care physicians and emergency physicians, this term raises a red flag for an acute coalescent mastoiditis, which is an otorhinolaryngological emergency. Unnecessary ear, nose, and throat (ENT) consultations are obtained to chase this radiological finding and inappropriate use of antibiotics can result.

To summarize, in the absence of bony erosion, subperiosteal abscesses, supportive clinical evidence, or in patients who are intubated, it is better to avoid the term mastoiditis for the radiological finding of mastoid opacification, and instead, the phrase "mastoid opacification please correlate clinically " should be used.[6–8]

Otomastoid Opacification Not Related to Inflammatory Disease

Although most cases of mastoid opacification are inflammatory, there are other entities in specific clinical scenarios that should prompt the search for other causes for this finding. In a previous prospective study, serous otitis media was found in 41% of patients with nasopharyngeal carcinoma. Nasopharyngeal carcinoma can be clinically silent and small; however, when it extends into the eustachian tube, it can present with hearing loss and serous otitis.[9] Therefore, in every adult with history of serous otitis, careful inspection of the nasopharynx should be performed to detect small nasopharyngeal carcinomas (**Fig. 7**).

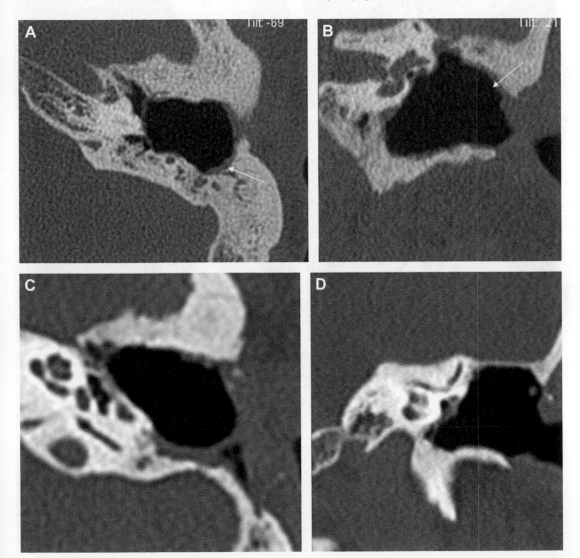

Fig. 10. Automastoidectomy versus surgical mastoidectomy. Axial and coronal CT images (*A, B*) demonstrate a cavity in the left mastoid air cells with a thin rim of peripheral soft tissue lining. This represents the so-called mural cholesteatoma shell in patient who has undergone auto mastoidectomy. Appearance is similar to a surgical defect created from a canal wall down mastoidectomy (*C, D*).

Patients with cerebrospinal fluid (CSF) otorrhea can also present with conductive hearing loss because of opacification of the mastoid air cells and middle ear. This may be post-traumatic or represent so-called spontaneous CSF leak from underlying idiopathic intracranial hypertension.[10] Many of these patients present with clear watery discharge from the nose or ear. CT scan of the temporal bone can reveal thinning or dehiscence of the tegmen and prominent arachnoid granulations along the anterior and posterior petrous ridge with osteodural defects (**Fig. 8**). Meningoceles and encephaloceles can also be seen, for which MRI is a better imaging modality (**Fig. 9**) Other signs of idiopathic intracranial hypertension can be seen in these cases, including a partially empty sella, prominence of the Meckel cave, prominent arachnoid granulations in the sphenoid wing, and increase perioptic CSF (see **Fig. 9**).

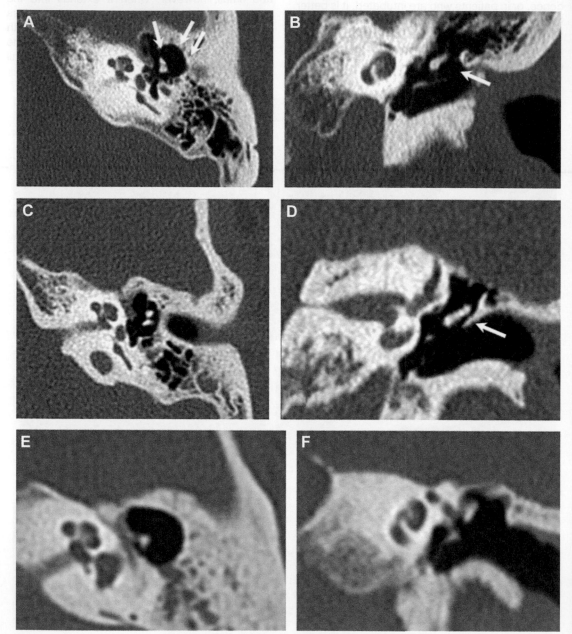

Fig. 11. Autoatticotomy versus surgical atticotomy. Axial and coronal CT (*A, B*) demonstrate widening (*arrow*) of the lateral attic on the axial images and absent scutum (*arrow*) on the coronal images. Compare that to a normal CT scan (*C, D*), which demonstrates normal dimension of the lateral attic and sharp scutum. (*E, F*) demonstrate a surgical atticotomy for localized attic cholesteatoma. The appearance is similar to the autoatticotomy cavity.

Apparent Postsurgical Appearance of the Temporal Bone -Automastoidectomy and Autoatticotomy

Cholesteatoma represents accumulation of keratinizing squamous epithelium in the middle ear cleft or other pneumatized portions of the temporal bone. It consists of a metabolically active outer lining of keratinizing squamous epithelium resulting in bony erosion. Centrally, it is composed of exfoliated acellular keratin debris secreted by the lining epithelium. In its acquired form, it is commonly seen in the pars flaccida and epitympanum as a result of eustachian tube dysfunction.

Automastoidectomy represents external evacuation of the contents of a cholesteatoma without operative intervention, creating the appearance of a surgical cavity. There is usually a smooth-walled cavity with destruction of the posterior wall of the EAC and exteriorization of the middle ear and mastoid. Sometimes, the bony cavity can be lined by the outer membrane of the original cholesteatoma with evacuation of the central keratin debris. In this instance, it is referred to as mural cholesteatoma shell (Fig. 10)

Autoatticotomy is a less extensive process of cholesteatoma autoevacuation in which the scutum is eroded and there is expansion of the lateral attic.[11] This mimics the appearance of a surgical atticotomy performed for limited attic cholesteatomas, especially when not accompanied by residual cholesteatoma (Fig. 11).

Bell Palsy versus Other Causes of Facial Nerve Paralysis

Bell palsy is the most common cause of facial nerve paralysis. It has been linked to herpes simplex virus type 1 infection reactivation in the geniculate ganglion. On imaging, enhancement of the labyrinthine segment of the facial nerve is most commonly seen in this disease process (Fig. 12). Other inflammatory causes of facial nerve paralysis include Lyme disease and sarcoid. Most patients with Bell palsy have complete spontaneous recovery within 6 months. However, if there is atypical clinical presentation, imaging is essential to exclude the possibility of neoplastic etiologies of facial nerve paralysis. This includes entities like schwannoma and perineural spread of neoplasm.[12] Perineural invasion can be seen in the setting of cutaneous squamous cell carcinomas and parotid malignancies like adenoid cystic carcinoma and muco-epidermoid carcinoma. Evaluation of the parotid should be performed in all patients who present with facial nerve symptoms to detect a possible source of perineural invasion (Fig. 13).

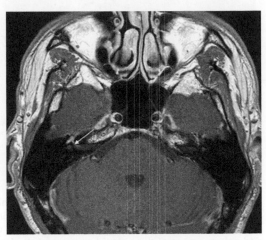

Fig. 12. Bell palsy. Axial poscontrast image demonstrates enhancement of the labyrinthine and geniculate segments of the right facial nerve (arrow). Findings resolved on follow-up imaging.

Sometimes, a patent facial nerve canal and meningocele of the geniculate fossa can be noted on imaging. On MRI, these lesions demonstrate prominent fluid along the labyrinthine segment of the facial nerve and fluid-filled remodeling and enlargement of the geniculate fossa (Fig. 14). On CT, similar appearance of the enlarged labyrinthine facial nerve canal and geniculate fossa is noted, with smooth expansile appearance. Although these findings may be associated with CSF otorrhea, meningitis, or facial paralysis, these fallopian canal meningoceles can also be incidental findings.[13]

Pulsatile Tinnitus Causes That May be Subtle on Imaging

Tinnitus is a sound in the ear, such as buzzing, ringing, or whistling, occurring without external stimulus. When it represents vascular sounds (both arterial or venous), it is referred to as pulsatile tinnitus (PT). The evaluation of a patient with tinnitus requires a detailed history, neuro-otologic physical examination with otoscopy, a comprehensive audiologic evaluation with hearing thresholds, and imaging studies. Multidetector CT (MDCT) of the temporal bone with contrast is the initial imaging modality of choice, and may be supplemented by CTA or MRI/magnetic resonance angiography (MRA)/magnetic resonance venography (MRV).

Sigmoid sinus dehiscence refers to a defect in the sigmoid sinus plate with lack of bony covering between the sigmoid sinus and the mastoid air cells.[14] It is among the most common identifiable causes of pulsatile tinnitus of venous origin.

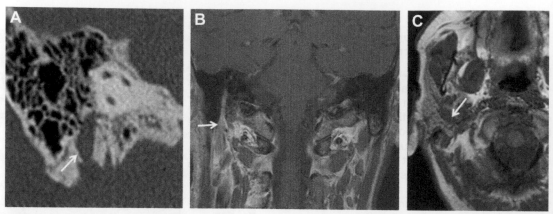

Fig. 13. Perineural invasion along the facial nerve. This patient presented with fully progressive facial paralysis on the right. On the coronal CT scan (*A*), subtle widening (*arrow*) of the mastoid segment of the facial nerve was seen, and an MRI was recommended. Coronal post gadolinoum MRI of the IAC (*B*) demonstrates enlargement and enhancement of the mastoid segment of the facial nerve extending down to the stylomastoid foramen (*arrow*). On the axial T1-weighted image (*C*), there is a mass in the right parotid gland. Pathology revealed adenoid cystic carcinoma of the parotid gland.

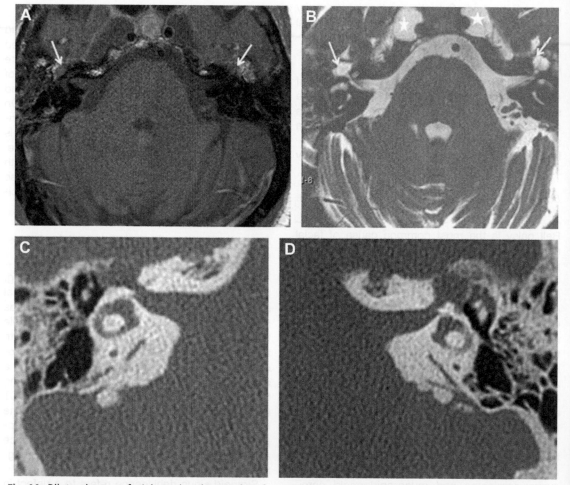

Fig. 14. Bilateral patent facial canal and geniculate fossa meningoceles. Axial postcontrast T1 weighted image (*A*) and axial 3-dimensional FIESTA image (*B*) through the IAC demonstrates cystic dilation of the geniculate ganglion bilaterally. On the axial 3-dimensional FIESTA image, bilateral enlargement of the Meckel cave is also seen (*star*). Corresponding findings on CT scan (*C, D*) of the temporal bone demonstrate characteristic bilateral bulbous dilation of the geniculate fossa.

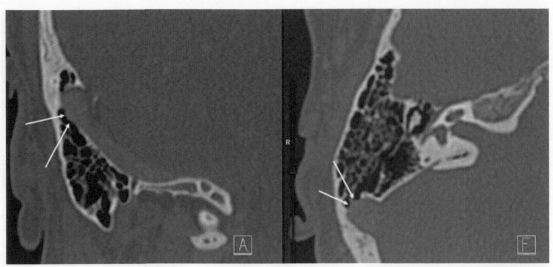

Fig. 15. Sigmoid sinus dehiscence. Coronal and axial CT image of the temporal bone in a patient with pulsatile tinnitus demonstrates lack of bony coverage of the sigmoid sinus in a short segment (*arrows*). This finding may be subtle and should be sought for any in a patient who presents with tinnitus.

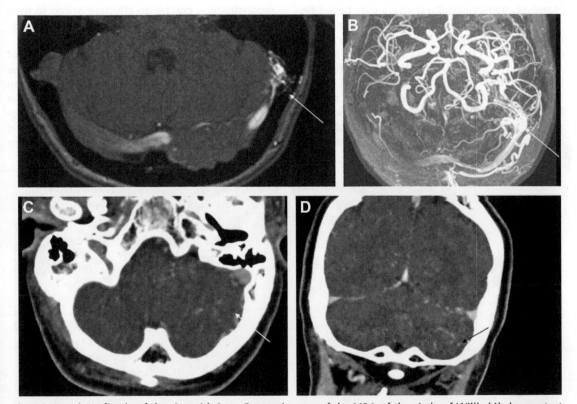

Fig. 16. Dural AV fistula of the sigmoid sinus. Source images of the MRA of the circle of Willis (*A*) demonstrate prominent signal in the left sigmoid sinus with transosseous collaterals (*arrows*). On the collapsed view of the MRA (*B*), asymmetric prominence of the left transverse sigmoid sinuses and multiple collateral vessels is noted. Axial and coronal CT images of the brain with contrast (*C, D*) demonstrate prominent serpiginous vessels in the posterior fossa in the different patient. This may be the earliest finding in patients with dural AV fistula and requires a high index of suspicion.

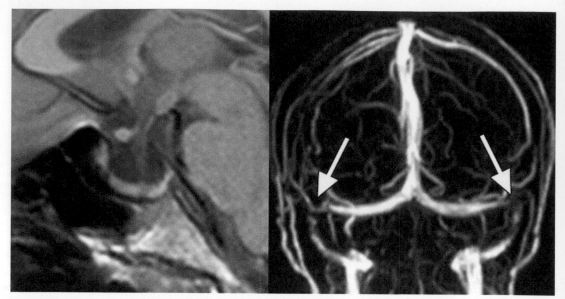

Fig. 17. Bilateral transverse sinus stenosis in a patient with pulsatile tinnitus caused by idiopathic intracranial hypertension. Sagittal T1-weighted image demonstrates an empty sella. MRV shows bilateral transverse sinus stenosis (*arrows*).

However, sometimes the findings may be subtle, and can be missed if not part of the search pattern in the setting of tinnitus. CT demonstrates a bony defect between the mastoid air cells and the sigmoid sinus, which may be in the anterior or anterolateral border of the superior curve or the descending segment of the sigmoid sinus.[15] Many of these patients may also have associated sigmoid sinus diverticulum (**Fig. 15**). In significantly symptomatic patients, sigmoid sinus wall reconstruction can be an effective option to treat pulsatile tinnitus with resurfacing of the dehiscence with bone cement.

PT may be the initial presenting symptom of dural atrioventricular (AV) fistula of the transverse sigmoid sinus. It represents an acquired lesion and may occur as a result of previous dural venous sinus thrombosis with revascularization. On cross-sectional imaging, the findings may be subtle and require a high index of suspicion. It is important to

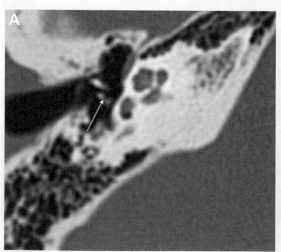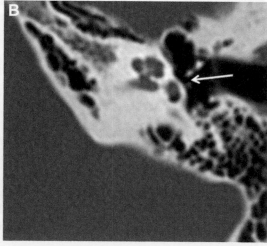

Fig. 18. Incudo-stapedial dislocation. Axial CT image of the right temporal bone (*A*) demonstrates normal incudostapedial joint (*arrow*). Axial CT image of the left temporal bone (*B*) shows a gap between the distal long process of the incus and the head of the stapes (*arrow*). This may be a subtle finding but should be part of one's checklist in the setting of conductive hearing loss.

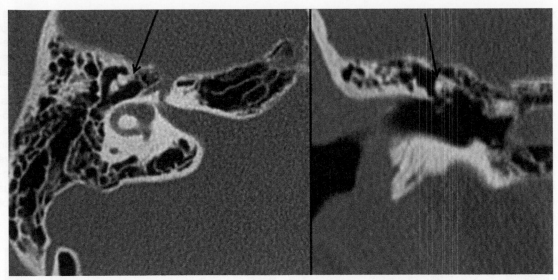

Fig. 19. Malleus fixation bar. Axial and coronal CT images demonstrate an osseous fixation bar (*arrow*) between the head of the malleus and the anterior epitympanum in a patient who presented with conductive hearing loss.

scrutinize the images carefully for signs of dural AV fistula, since this is potentially a curable cause of tinnitus. These findings include enlarged and tortuous vessels in the posterior fossa and enlarged transosseous channels. Magnetic resonance angiogram shows arterialization of flow in the venous sinuses and external carotid arterial feeders are identified (**Fig. 16**).The collapsed view of MRA will reveal asymmetric prominence of vasculature at the sigmoid transverse sinus junction on one side and is a useful image to obtain. Catheter angiogram is the gold standard for diagnosis, classification, and treatment.

Another common cause of tinnitus is idiopathic intracranial hypertension (IIH). Transverse sinus stenosis in patients with idiopathic intracranial hypertension can contribute to tinnitus (**Fig. 17**), and all patients who present with tinnitus should be examined for imaging findings of idiopathic intracranial hypertension including empty sella, prominent Meckel cave, increased CSF surrounding tortuous optic sheaths, and prominent arachnoid granulations in the sphenoid wing and the petrous ridge.

Conductive Hearing Loss in the Setting of a Normal Tympanic Membrane

Conductive hearing loss is caused by interference in the transmission of sound energy from the

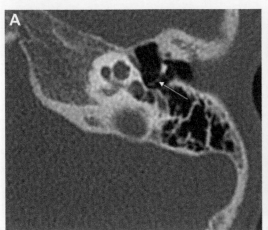
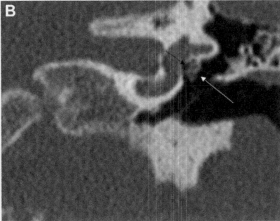

Fig. 20. Congenital anomalies of the ossicles, facial nerve, and oval window. Axial and coronal CT images demonstrate dysmorphic appearance of the stapes with a normal posterior crura (*arrow* in *A*) and poorly defined anterior crus. Coronal CT images demonstrate dehiscent facial nerve onto the stapes (*white arrow*). Oval window stenosis is also seen (*black arrow*). This patient presented with congenital conductive hearing loss.

external environment through the external auditory canal, middle ear cavity, and onto the oval window. Many of the lesions that result in conductive hearing loss may be evident clinically to the otologist and radiologist, including cholesteatoma, otomastoiditis or glomus tumor. CT is the main imaging modality used to assess patients with conductive hearing loss.

There are several subtle causes of conductive hearing loss that may not be readily apparent on first glance on a temporal bone CT. As such, an organized approach and systematic evaluation of important anatomic structures is required to ensure that lesions are not missed. Otosclerosis has already been discussed. Ossicular chain abnormalities can also be missed on initial evaluation, because they are not part of the pattern of search of the radiologist. Because of improvements in imaging technique and resolution, the ossicles can be optimally visualized in greater anatomic detail. Sagittal or Poschl views are especially useful in assessing anatomy of the ossicles. Ossicular lesions include incudo-stapedial dislocation (post-traumatic) (**Fig. 18**), congenital dysmorphic ossicles with osseous defects, fixation bars (**Fig. 19**), and dehiscence of the facial nerve into the oval window or stapes (**Fig. 20**). Resorption of the distal long process of the incus (**Fig. 21**) may be related to congenital causes or postinflammatory hyperemic changes.

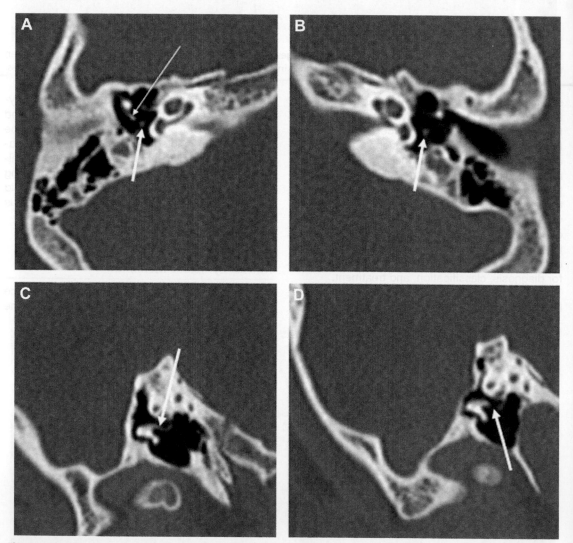

Fig. 21. Erosion of the distal long process of the incus. On the right, there is normal appearance (A) of the distal long process of the incus (*long arrow*) and the head of the stapes (*arrow*). The normal distal long process is seen to good advantage on the sagittal CT image (*arrow* in C). Conversely, on the left, although the head of the stapes is seen (*arrow* in B), the distal long process of the incus is not visualized on either the axial or the sagittal image (B, D).

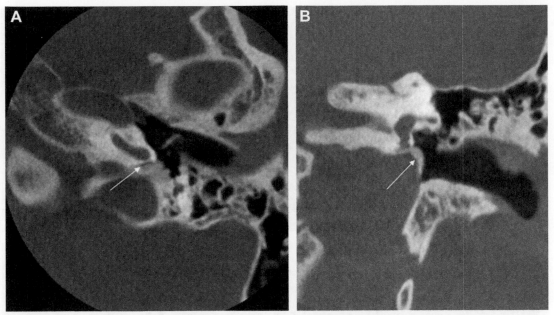

Fig. 22. Round window occlusion by an osteoma. Axial (*A*) and coronal (*B*) CT images demonstrate an osseous lesion arising from the hypotympanum, occluding the round window. On otoscopy, this appeared like a white mass, and the clinical question was cholesteatoma. These patients can present with conductive hearing loss because of occlusion of the round window.

Finally, round window occlusion/stenosis can also present with conductive hearing loss because of an increase in the resistance to acoustic energy entering the cochlea. Some causes of round window stenosis include congenital stenosis, inflammation, bony lesions (**Fig. 22**), and high riding jugular bulb or jugular bulb diverticulum (**Fig. 23**).

The round window area should be on the radiologist's checklist in addition to ossicular chain abnormalities as mentioned previously. Jugular bulb vascular lesions can also result in inadvertent injury on tympanoplasty and should be pointed out in the radiology report, especially in the preoperative setting (see **Fig. 23**).

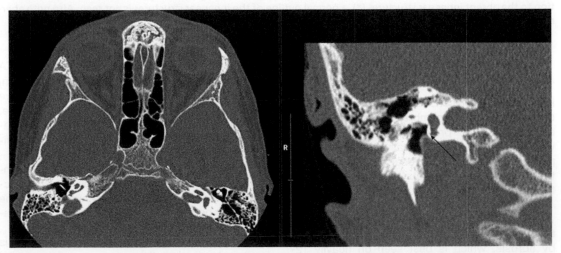

Fig. 23. Diverticulum of the jugular bulb. Axial and coronal CT images demonstrate diverticulum of the right jugular bulb, which projects into the hypotympanum and obstructs the round window (*arrow*). This is also an important finding in a preoperative setting.

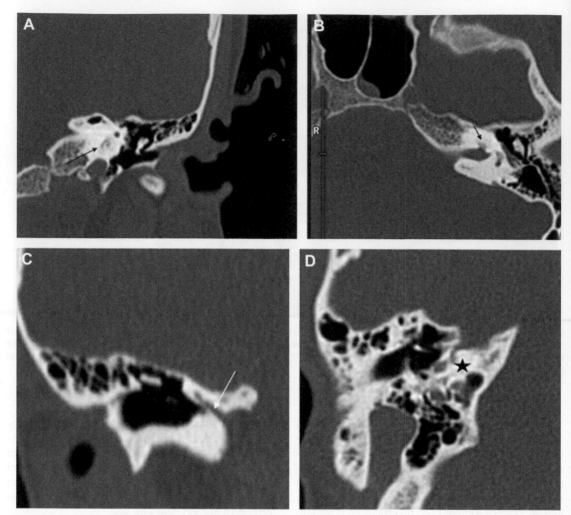

Fig. 24. Severe labyrinthitis ossificans. Axial and coronal CT images (*A, B*) demonstrate markedly sclerotic appearance of the left cochlea and to a lesser extent the vestibule. However, the outline of a normal cochlea is seen on both images (*arrows*). In contradistinction to this, in a patient with congenital labyrinthine aplasia (*C, D*), in addition to the absent inner ear structures (*), a normal outline of the inner ear structures is not seen. Also note aberrant course of the facial nerve (*arrow* in *C*), which may be seen in congenital anomalies of the inner ear.

Severe Labyrinthitis Ossificans versus Labyrinthine Aplasia

Labyrinthitis ossificans (LO) refers to ossification of the lumen of the membranous labyrinth and is associated with profound hearing loss and vestibular dysfunction, usually as a sequela of prior inflammation (bacterial meningitis being the most common cause). Other causes include trauma, hemorrhage or autoimmune disease. Acute labyrinthitis presents as enhancement within the structures of the labyrinth on postcontrast images. The subacute stage is manifested by fibrosis, which is best seen on heavily T2-weighted sequences through the internal auditory canal (IAC) including constructive

interference in steady state (CISS) or FIESTA (fast imaging employing steady-state acquisition) sequences.[16] These 2 stages of labyrinthitis are occult on CT. Later in the course of the disease, there is high density noted within the membranous labyrinth on CT scan, which is the ossificans stage of the inflammation (**Fig. 24**A, B).

The treatment for hearing loss related to labyrinthitis is cochlear implantation. However, the success of the procedure is much higher when the surgery is performed before the fibrous or ossification stage has set in, which is best seen on MRI.

Sometimes, when the labyrinthitis ossificans is severe, it can mimic the appearance of congenital labyrinthine aplasia (**Fig. 24**C, D). In labyrinthitis ossificans, this shape and contour of the labyrinth are preserved, but not in patients with congenital labyrinthine aplasia.

CLINICS CARE POINTS

- Radiologists should familiarize themselves with expected CT appearance of temporal bone sutures, channels and fissures to avoid calling them fractures.

- Mastoiditis is a clinical term and should not be used routinely in radiology reports for opacified air cells without osseous erosion.

- Besides inflammatory disease, CSF lead can be a cause of opacified mastoid air cells. The images should be examined for other imaging findings of idiopathic intracranial hypertension.

- Ossicular fixation and inflammatory resorption of the incus long process may be a subtle finding on CT temporal bone and detailed evaluation of the ossicles should be performed in patients who present with conductive hearing loss.

DISCLOSURE

The authors have nothing to disclose.

REFERENCES

1. Kwong Y, Yu D, Shah J. Fracture mimics on temporal bone CT: a guide for the radiologist. AJR Am J Roentgenol 2012;199(2):428–34.

2. Koesling S, Kunkel P, Schul T. Vascular anomalies, sutures and small canals of the temporal bone on axial CT. Eur J Radiol 2005;54:335–43.

3. Chadwell JB, Halsted MJ, Choo DI, et al. The cochlear cleft. AJNR Am J Neuroradiol 2004;25: 21–24.

4. Sanverdi SE, Ozgen B, Dolgun A, et al. Incomplete endochondral ossification of the otic capsule, a variation in children: evaluation of its prevalence and extent in children with and without sensorineural hearing loss. AJNR Am J Neuroradiol 2015;36(1): 171–5.

5. Milroy CM, Michaels L. Pathology of the otic capsule. J Laryngol Otol 1990;104:83–90.

6. Sayal NR, Boyd S, Zach White G, et al. Incidental mastoid effusion diagnosed on imaging: are we doing right by our patients? Laryngoscope 2019;129: 852–7.

7. Pastuszek, A et al. "Is mastoiditis being over-diagnosed on computed tomography imaging? —radiological versus clinical findings." 2020. Available at: https://www.theajo.com/article/view/4325/html.

8. McDonald MH, Hoffman MR, Gentry LR. When is fluid in the mastoid cells a worrisome finding? J Am Board Fam Med 2013;26(2):218–20.

9. Sham JST, Wei WI, Lau SK, et al. Serous otitis media: an opportunity for early recognition of nasopharyngeal carcinoma. Arch Otolaryngol Head Neck Surg 1992;118(8):794–7.

10. Bidot S, Levy JM, Saindane AM, et al. Do most patients with a spontaneous cerebrospinal fluid leak have idiopathic intracranial hypertension? J Neuroophthalmol 2019;39(4):487–95.

11. Manasawala M, Cunnane ME, Curtin HD, et al. Imaging findings in auto-atticotom. Am J Neuroradiology 2014;35(1):182–5.

12. Quesnel AM, Lindsay RW, Hadlock TA. When the bell tolls on Bell's palsy: finding occult malignancy in acute-onset facial paralysis. Am J Otolaryngol 2010;31(5):339–42.

13. Benson JC, Krecke K, Geske JR, et al. Prevalence of spontaneous asymptomatic facial nerve canal meningoceles: a retrospective review. AJNR Am J Neuroradiol 2019;40(8):1402–5.

14. Lansley JA, Tucker W, Eriksen MR, et al. Sigmoid sinus diverticulum, dehiscence, and venous sinus stenosis: potential causes of pulsatile tinnitus in patients with idiopathic intracranial hypertension? AJNR Am J Neuroradiol 2017;38(9):1783–8.

15. Geng W, Liu Z, Fan Z. CT characteristics of dehiscent sigmoid plates presenting as pulsatile tinnitus: a study of 23 patients. Acta Radiol 2015;56(11): 1404–8.

16. Booth TN, Roland P, Kutz JW, et al. High-resolution 3-D T2-weighted imaging in the diagnosis of labyrinthitis ossificans: emphasis on subtle cochlear involvement. Pediatr Radiol 2013;43(12):1584–90.

Normal Anatomic Structures and Variants of the Sinonasal Cavities, Orbit, and Jaw

Gul Moonis, MD

KEYWORDS

• Mucocele • Polyp • Sinonasal organized hematoma • Odontogenic sinusitis

KEY POINTS

• There are important anatomic variants in the sinonasal cavity that can increase the risk of iatrogenic injury during surgery and should be looked for in all preoperative studies.
• There may be overlap in MR imaging features of benign and malignant polyps. Bony destruction on computed tomographic (CT) scan will be a helpful sign to differentiate these.
• Hyperostotic stalk is a useful feature seen on sinonasal CT in cases of inverting papilloma.
• Sinusitis can be related to odontogenic causes, and all cases of sinonasal inflammation should have the dentition closely scrutinized for potential dental cause.

SINONASAL ANATOMIC VARIANTS POSING POTENTIAL SURGICAL HAZARD

Functional endoscopic sinus surgery is a common surgical method for treatment of chronic rhinosinusitis. Preoperative imaging is essential to guide surgery. Several variants of the paranasal sinuses are of primary importance in surgical planning.[1] An important sinonasal variant that can present a potential surgical hazard is dehiscence of the cribriform plate. This increases the risk of iatrogenic intracranial entry. A deep olfactory fossa with thin lateral lamella of the cribriform plate (Keros classification 3) increases risk of iatrogenic intracranial entry (**Fig. 1**) and can also be a site of erosions related to meningoencephalocele. Similarly, dehiscence of the lamina papyracea should be noted on preoperative imaging to decrease the possibility of intraorbital injury of surgical instruments. The presence of an Onodi air cell (sphenoethmoidal air cell) in which a posterior ethmoid air cell extends posteriorly along the superior and lateral aspect of the sphenoid sinus is an important variant, as the optic nerve courses through this air cell. This can increase the risk of optic nerve injury during surgery. This air cell is best visualized on coronal images (see **Fig. 1**B).

The relative position of the anterior ethmoidal artery with respect to the skull base should be noted. The artery is said to be unprotected if there is aeration between it and the skull base. If the artery is at the level of the skull base, it is in a protected position (**Fig. 2**). To decrease iatrogenic injury to the optic nerve or the carotid canal, the presence or absence of bony coverage of these structures should be noted.

BENIGN VERSUS MALIGNANT SINONASAL SOFT TISSUE

On noncontrast sinonasal computed tomographic (CT) scan, which is the initial imaging study for sinus symptoms, one often sees polypoid soft tissue within the nasal cavity, and it can be difficult to distinguish inflammatory polypoid mucosal thickening from tumor. In addition, sinonasal tumors often lead to coexisting inflammatory change, as they obstruct drainage pathways. For these

Department of Radiology, NYU Langone Medical Center, 222 E 41st Street, New York, NY 10017, USA
E-mail address: gul.moonis@nyulangone.org

Neuroimag Clin N Am 32 (2022) 363–374
https://doi.org/10.1016/j.nic.2022.01.008

neuroimaging.theclinics.com

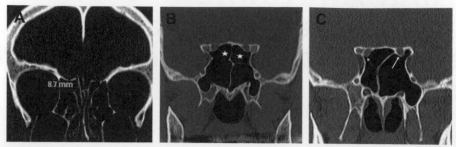

Fig. 1. Important sinonasal anatomic variants closing potential surgical hazard. (A) Coronal CT image through the anterior skull base demonstrates a deep olfactory fossa on the right measuring 8.7 mm. This can predispose to iatrogenic intracranial entry. (B) Coronal CT image through the sphenoid sinus demonstrates bilateral Onodi air cells (*asterisk*) superior to the sphenoid sinus. The optic nerve when traveling through this air cell is at risk of contiguous spread of infection. (C) Coronal CT image demonstrates dehiscence of the right bony canal of the optic nerve (*thin arrow*). The left bony canal is intact (*thick arrow*). The intersinus septum of the sphenoid sinus inserts on the left optic canal, another point to note in CT sinus performed for pre-surgical planning.

reasons, interpretation must take into account findings that can herald more serious pathologic condition.

A mildly expansile mass most commonly arising from the maxillary sinus, extending into the nasal cavity with internal speckled hyperdensity, can represent either a fungus ball with inflammatory obstruction, an inverted papilloma, or an antrochoanal polyp. On CT scan, the fungus ball is a high-density mass with calcifications and surrounding circumferential hypoattenuating mucosal thickening. Bony margins are intact. On MR imaging, a fungus ball is hypointense on T2-weighted images and isointense to hypointense on T1-weighted images. Postgadolinium images usually demonstrate enhancement of the surrounding inflammatory mucosa (Fig. 3).

Inverted papillomas are benign sinonasal tumors arising from Schneiderian mucosa and are associated with human papillomavirus infection. On CT scan, the lesion presents as a lobulated sinus mass without aggressive erosion. A hyperostotic stalk is useful sign seen on CT scan and is thought to represent its site of origin (Fig. 4A, B). On MR imaging, a convoluted cerebriform appearance is noted on T2-weighted and postgadolinium images (Fig. 4C).

An antrochoanal polyp is a benign solitary polyp arising in most cases from the maxillary sinus via a narrow stalk. It is seen more frequently in children

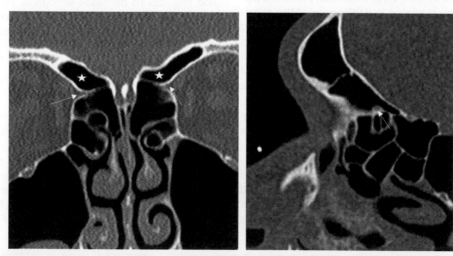

Fig. 2. Unprotected course of the anterior ethmoidal artery. Coronal and sagittal CT images of the paranasal sinuses demonstrate pneumatization (*asterisk*) superior to the anterior ethmoidal arteries bilaterally (*arrows*). The artery travels in a mesentery direction rather than being flush against the skull base. In this configuration, the artery is at risk for iatrogenic injury.

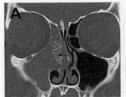
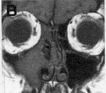
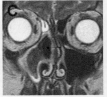
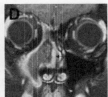

Fig. 3. Fungus ball. Coronal CT scan (*A*) of the paranasal sinuses demonstrates a lesion with speckled calcifications at the right lateral nasal wall (*arrow*) with secondary obstruction of right maxillary and ethmoid sinuses. Coronal T1- (*B*) and T2-weighted (*C*) images demonstrate the lesion to be hypointense (*arrow*). Note the obstructed secretions in the right maxillary sinus, which are hypointense on the T2-weighted images (*star*) but less so than the fungus ball. This is because the fungus ball is calcified, whereas the obstructed secretions are inspissated. Postgadolinium images (*D*) demonstrate circumferential mucosal enhancement of the sinus (*arrow*).

than adults. Macroscopically, it demonstrates a cystic intramaxillary portion and a solid intranasal portion. On CT scan, it can be low or high density (if associated with proteinaceous secretions or fungal colonization). There is characteristic widening of the maxillary ostium and lack of aggressive bony destruction (**Fig. 5**). On MR imaging, it follows water signal on T1- and T2-weighted images, unless it is proteinaceous, in which case it will demonstrate areas of increased T1 and intermediate to decreased T2 signal intensity. After administration of contrast, there may be a thin rim of mucosal enhancement. However, the central portion of the polyp does not enhance.

Aggressive-appearing, permeative bony destruction may be seen in the setting of squamous cell carcinoma, the most common sinonasal malignancy. Any polypoid lesion with this pattern of bone destruction should raise concern for malignancy. On MR imaging, malignancies are usually isointense to hypointense on T2-weighted images with restricted diffusion (**Fig. 6**), and benign lesions are T2 hyperintense. It should be noted however that some benign inflammatory polyps can have overlapping appearance with malignancy on MR

imaging (**Fig. 7**). In these cases, nonaggressive CT pattern of bony erosion might be helpful in differentiation.

Meningoencephaloceles of the anterior and central skull base can be congenital or acquired and may mimic a polypoid mass on CT scan, but the bony defect has a nonaggressive appearance (**Fig. 8A**). Look for other signs of idiopathic intracranial hypertension in acquired anterior and central skull-base meningoencephaloceles (**Fig. 8B–D**). These include partially empty sella, tortuous and enlarged optic nerve sheaths, enlarged Meckel caves, and prominent arachnoid pits. If there is isolated opacification of a single or few sinuses, cerebrospinal fluid leak should be excluded both clinically and on imaging.

Normal sinus secretions are watery and appear hypointense on T1-weighted images and hyperintense on T2-weighted images. As sinus secretions become more dense and inspissated, particularly with superimposed fungal colonization, the protein concentration increases, which can result in hyperintense signal on T1-weighted images and hypointense signal/signal void on T2-weighted image. In these cases, they will appear aerated on

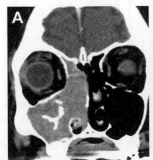
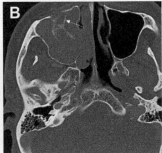
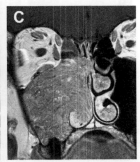

Fig. 4. Inverted papilloma. Coronal and axial CT scan of the right maxillary sinus demonstrate an expansile lesion in the right maxillary sinus with extension to the ethmoid air cells (*A, B*). On the axial bone windows, noted is the hyperostotic stalk (*arrow*), which is characteristic of this lesion. On the coronal postgadolinium images, characteristic convoluted cerebriform appearance of the lesion is seen (*C*). Also noted to better advantage on the MR imaging is that the lesion expands the inferior orbital wall but does not violate the periorbita.

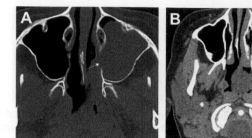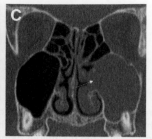

Fig. 5. Antrochoanal polyp. Axial (*A, B*) and coronal (*C*) images from a sinus CT scan demonstrate a polypoid lesion extending from the left maxillary sinus into the nasopharyngeal lumen through an expanded maxillary sinus ostium (*arrow* in *A* and *C*). On the axial soft tissue windows (*B*), the large nasopharyngeal component of the lesion is seen (*star*).

MR images, despite being filled with thick secretions. This is the so-called pseudoaerated appearance of paranasal sinuses on MR imaging (**Fig. 9**). If there is a discrepancy between the clinical presentation and the findings on MR imaging, noncontrast CT scan will demonstrate the actual pathologic condition. On postcontrast examinations, what may initially appear to be an enhancing mass lesion, may, on review of the precontrast images, simply be a nonenhancing mucocele (**Fig. 10**).

Mucoceles of the paranasal sinuses occur because of obstruction of the sinus ostium. Over time, pressure builds up within the sinus, resulting in remodeling and expansion of the sinus walls, which may press into adjacent structures like the orbit and brain. On CT scan, mucoceles appear as completely opacified sinuses with smooth bony expansion of the walls. There is no frank bony destruction as would be seen with more aggressive lesions, such as sinonasal cancer. On MR imaging, owing to the

heterogeneous appearance of sinus secretions, the mucocele can be bright on T1-weighted images and hypointense on T2-weighted images. Although most mucoceles are inflammatory, be aware that an obstructing mass/neoplasm can also result in a mucocele (**Fig. 11**). Sinus expansion can also be seen in the setting of cystic bony neoplasms like aneurysmal bone cysts (ABCs). ABCs are expansile blood-filled channels that can be either primary or secondary. There are multiple theories as to their cause, including trauma, altered hemodynamic state, or secondary to a preexisting bony lesion (chondroblastoma, giant cell tumor, or fibrous dysplasia).[2] The primary osseous lesion is thought to initiate an osseous arteriovenous fistula through which hemodynamic forces create a secondary reactive lesion, such as an ABC. There may be rapid growth of the lesion, and patients may present with acute symptoms; in this clinical scenario, development of secondary ABC should be considered (**Fig. 12**).

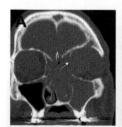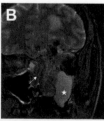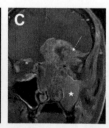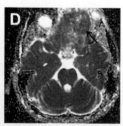

Fig. 6. Sinonasal undifferentiated carcinoma of the ethmoid sinus. Coronal CT image (*A*) of the sinus demonstrates a large soft tissue lesion in the ethmoid sinus, maxillary sinus, and nasal cavity with intraorbital extension (*white arrow*). Erosion of the cribriform plate is also seen (*black arrow*). MR images help to demarcate the true margins of this lesion. Coronal T2-weighted image demonstrates the T2 iso-hypointense signal of this lesion, which is characteristic for sinonasal malignancies. Intracranial (*white arrow* in *C*) and intraorbital (*black arrow* in *C*) extensions are better seen than on the CT scan. MR imaging also helps differentiate obstructed secretions (*asterisk* in *B* and *C*) from neoplasm. Obstructed secretions tend to be hyperintense on T2-weighted images and isointense to hyperintense on T1-weighted images owing to the presence of protein. ADC map (*D*) demonstrates restricted diffusion (*arrow*) within this lesion, which is characteristic of malignancies.

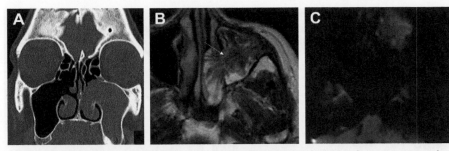

Fig. 7. Antrochoanal polyp. Coronal CT image (*A*) through the paranasal sinuses demonstrates a classic polypoid lesion extending from the maxillary sinus into the nasal cavity through an expanded maxillary sinus ostium. MR imaging in this case was not as straightforward. Coronal T2-weighted image (*B*) demonstrates striations (*arrow*) reminiscent of convoluted cerebriform appearance seen in Inverted Papilloma. Restricted diffusion is seen on diffusion-weighted images (*C*) related to proteinaceous content. This case underscores the fact that sometimes MR imaging appearance of inflammatory polyps may be confusing and may mimic neoplasm.

SINONASAL ORGANIZED HEMATOMA

Sinonasal organized hematoma is a nonneoplastic hemorrhagic lesion of the maxillary sinus. It consists of a chronic hematoma with a surrounding organized fibrous capsule, related to prior repeated hemorrhages with subsequent encapsulation. Encapsulation prevents the resorption of the hematoma and induces neovascularization with further bouts of bleeding. This results in progressive expansion and local bony demineralization. Predisposing factors include trauma, sinus surgery, radiation infections, or bleeding diathesis. On noncontrast CT scan, these lesions are expansile and hypodense when compared with soft tissue but may contain areas of focal hyperattenuation. On T1-weighted images, these lesions are intermediate signal, and on T2-weighted images, the lesions are heterogeneously T2 hypointense with a peripheral hypointense rim, which corresponds to the fibrous pseudocapsule. There is patchy heterogeneous enhancement, which may be nodular, papillary, or frondlike (**Fig. 13**). This characteristic imaging feature helps in differentiating this lesion from malignancies.[3]

ROUNDED OPACITY IN THE MAXILLARY SINUS

Mucous retention cysts are common incidental imaging findings of the paranasal sinuses caused by obstruction of the seromucinous glands of the sinonasal mucosa. On imaging, these lesions appear as smooth, rounded soft tissue masses, hypoattenuating on CT scan images, hypointense on T1-weighted images, hyperintense on T2-weighted images without enhancement.

However, odontogenic cysts of both inflammatory and developmental origin (radicular cysts and dentigerous cysts among others) may have a similar imaging appearance with an apparent lucent lobulated lesion within the floor of the maxillary sinus. In many of these cases, a helpful sign is to look for a thin rim of bone along the superior aspect of the lesion or disease in the adjacent

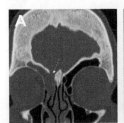
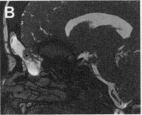
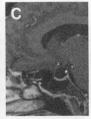
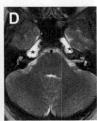

Fig. 8. Meningoencephalocele presenting as sinus disease. Coronal CT scan (*A*) of the paranasal sinuses demonstrates polypoid soft tissue density (*star*) in the right frontal and ethmoid sinuses, which was presumed to be inflammatory. However, a bony defect was seen in the roof of the right ethmoid sinus (*arrow*). On the sagittal FIESTA sequence (*B*), there is good demarcation between the encephalocele (*arrow*) and T2 hyperintense obstructive secretions in the frontal sinus. On sagittal postgadolinium image (*C*), there is an empty sella (*arrow*), and prominent Meckel caves are noted on the axial T2-weighted image (*stars* in *D*). This patient was eventually diagnosed with idiopathic intracranial hypertension.

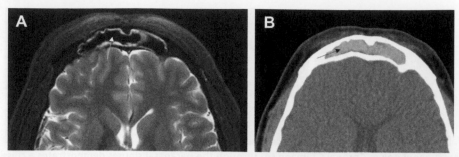

Fig. 9. Pseudo-aerated appearance of the frontal sinus. On the axial CT scan (B), the frontal sinus is filled with hyperdense secretions (arrow) in this patient with allergic fungal sinusitis. However, on the axial T2-weighted image (A), there is a deceptive aerated appearance of the central sinus (arrow) with only mild peripheral T2 hyperintensity. This is related to inspissation of the sinus secretions.

tooth, which points to the odontogenic origin of the lesion (Fig. 14).

SINUSITIS RELATED TO ODONTOGENIC CAUSES

Rhinosinusitis or chronic inflammation of the paranasal sinuses is a very common condition encountered clinically. Approximately 10% to 30% of sinusitis cases are related to the underlying odontogenic process. Odontogenic sinusitis refers to dental origin of this inflammation on the basis of either radiographic, microbiologic, or clinical evidence. Furthermore, iatrogenic causes like oroantral fistula following dental extract or dental implant surgery may also be associated with an increased iatrogenic risk of odontogenic sinusitis.[4] Failure to identify a dental cause can lead to recalcitrant sinusitis with potential for serious complications. On imaging, mucosal thickening in the floor of the maxillary sinus is seen with adjacent

periapical inflammatory changes usually in the maxillary molars, postdental extraction oral-antral fistula, or complications related to dental implants (Fig. 15).

SMALL SIZE OF MAXILLARY SINUS

Silent sinus syndrome, also known as chronic maxillary sinus atelectasis, consists of painless enophthalmos, hypoglobus, and inward retraction of the maxillary sinus walls on imaging. Longstanding obstruction of the maxillary sinus ostium/infundibulum is related to the development of silent sinus syndrome, and the condition is considered to be idiopathic. Because of maxillary sinus ostium occlusion, negative pressure is generated within the sinus leading to gradual inward bowing of all the maxillary sinus walls. The sinus itself is fully formed, unlike maxillary sinus hypoplasia, and is either partially or completely opacified.[5] The uncinate process is superolaterally

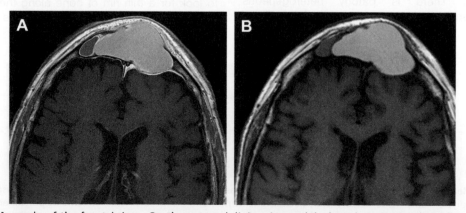

Fig. 10. Mucocele of the frontal sinus. On the postgadolinium image (A), there is an expansile T1 hyperintense mass in the frontal sinus. Initially, this was mistaken for an enhancing expansile neoplasm, and the patient was scheduled for surgery. Initially, the noncontrast T1-weighted images were not performed. Subsequently, a noncontrast T1-weighted image (B) demonstrates a classic proteinaceous frontal mucocele, which is intrinsically T1 hyperintense.

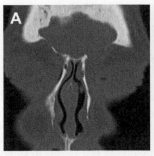
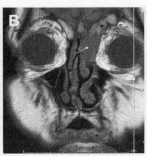
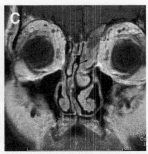

Fig. 11. Mucocele related to an underlying obstructive mass. Coronal CT (*A*) image demonstrates an expansile lesion of the frontal sinus with marked thinning/dehiscence of the sinus walls most suggestive of a mucocele. MR coronal images (T1-weighted images precontrast and postcontrast, *B* and *C*, respectively) demonstrate demarcation between an enhancing obstructive mass in the left ethmoid sinus (*arrows*) versus intrinsically T1 hyperintense proteinaceous secretions of the frontoethmoidal mucocele (*star* in *B*). Pathology revealed inverting papilloma.

displaced, and the ostiomeatal complex is occluded. There is enlargement of the middle meatus related to lateral retraction of the middle turbinate (**Fig. 16**A, B). Maxillary sinus hypoplasia can be unilateral or bilateral. The underlying cause is uncertain but is thought to be either developmental or related to sinusitis in the first years of life. Imaging criteria include elevated canine fossa and enlarged alveolar process of the maxillary sinus (**Fig. 16**C, D). Other findings that may be seen are an increase in the vertical dimension of the orbit, lateral position of the infraorbital nerve canal, and enlarged pterygopalatine fossa. The uncinate process is usually hypoplastic and lateralized, and the maxillary sinus is opacified.

OPACIFIED OLFACTORY CLEFT

Respiratory epithelial adenomatoid hamartoma (REAH) is a benign glandular neoplasm of the sinonasal cavities and is frequently found in the olfactory clefts.[6] On CT scan, it presents as a nonenhancing homogeneous mass with widening of the olfactory cleft (**Fig. 17**A). On MR imaging, findings are nonspecific with variable gadolinium enhancement. These imaging findings can mimic sinonasal polyposis or meningoencephalocele of the cribriform plate (**Fig. 17**B), although with meningocele, a defect of the cribriform plate would be seen. The importance of suggesting REAH in the differential diagnosis of olfactory cleft masses is to help prevent aggressive surgical procedures with increased risk of complications.

LUCENT MANDIBULAR LESION WITH NONAGGRESSIVE MARGINS

Stafne bone cavity is an incidental unilateral nonaggressive oval-shaped radiolucency in the posterior margin of the mandible below the mylohyoid line and above the inferior border of the mandible.[7] It is thought to be related to remodeling

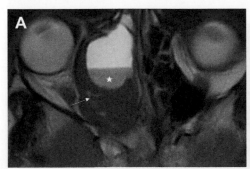
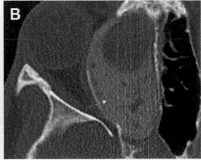

Fig. 12. Secondary ABC of the ethmoid sinus. MR scan was initially performed (*A*), which demonstrated a cystic lesion within the right ethmoid sinus with a hemorrhage fluid level (*star*). The right ethmoid air cells were replaced by a lesion, which was T2 hypointense (*arrow*). Gadolinium was not administered. CT scan axial image (*B*) performed later demonstrates a classic ground-glass appearance (*arrow*) of the ethmoid sinus compatible with fibrous dysplasia. This patient presented with worsening proptosis and right eye pain.

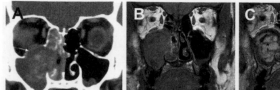
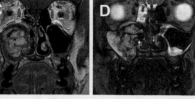

Fig. 13. Sinonasal organized hematoma. Coronal CT image without contrast (*A*) shows a heterogeneously hyperdense expansile lesion (*black arrows*) in the right maxillary sinus with thinning of the periorbita (*arrow*). Coronal T1-weighted (*B*), coronal postgadolinium T1-weighted image (*B*), and coronal T2-weighted image with fat saturation shows central enhancement (*star* in *C*) and characteristic T2 hypointense foci (*arrow* in *D*) seen with the lesion. Obstructed secretions are noted in the right ethmoid sinus (*star*) and right maxillary sinus.

of the mandibular cortex by pressure exerted by the submandibular gland. Most commonly seen in middle-aged men, this benign entity can be misdiagnosed as a lytic jaw lesion. Although some lesions may contain salivary tissue, many of the lesions may appear to contain only fat or nonspecific soft tissue (**Fig. 18**).

MIXED LYTIC SCLEROTIC LESIONS OF THE JAW

Medication-related osteonecrosis of the jaw (is clinically defined as exposed bone or bone present for more than 8 weeks that can be probed through a fistula in the mandible and maxilla.[8] It is a known side effect of antiangiogenic or antiresorptive medications. It is most commonly related to the use of bisphosphonates and denosumab. No history of radiation therapy or obvious metastatic lesions to the jaw should be present. On imaging, findings may be very similar to osteomyelitis or osteoradionecrosis with heterogeneous lytic sclerotic lesions with a sequestrum, periosteal reaction, cortical erosion, or soft tissue swelling (**Fig. 19**). Obtaining appropriate clinical history is critical to making this diagnosis.

EXTRAOCULAR MUSCLE ENLARGEMENT

Thyroid-associated orbitopathy is an autoimmune process related to dysthyroid states. Autoantibodies target the thyroid-stimulating hormone receptors on thyroid cells, resulting in excess of thyroid hormone. However, this entity can also be seen in euthyroid and hypothyroid patients. In addition to hyperthyroidism, many patients develop an orbitopathy characterized by deposition of glycosaminoglycan's, fibrosis of the extraocular muscles, and adipogenesis in the orbit. Although enlarged extraocular muscles in the orbit are related most commonly to thyroid orbitopathy, pseudotumor/idiopathic orbital inflammation can also have a similar presentation. The only difference is that the most common muscles involved with thyroid orbitopathy are superior rectus/levator palpebrae superioris complex, inferior rectus, and medial rectus, in that order, whereas with pseudotumor, the lateral rectus is the most commonly involved muscle (**Fig. 20**A, B). In addition, Graves disease tends to be bilateral versus pseudotumor, which is commonly unilateral. Other entities that can present with enlargement of the extraocular muscles include sarcoidosis, IgG4-related disease, and lymphoma. Sometimes,

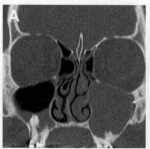
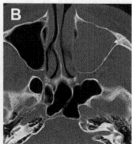
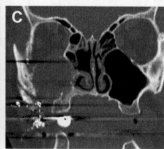

Fig. 14. Odontogenic cyst mimicking mucus retention cyst. Coronal (*A*) and axial (*B*) CT images show complete opacification of the left maxillary sinus. Initially, this was thought to represent a mucous retention cyst. However, the presence of a thin rim of bone along the superior aspect of the lesion (*arrow*) indicated an odontogenic origin. (*C*) There is an expansile lesion in the right maxillary sinus in this patient with prior facial trauma. This was a posttraumatic mucocele of the sinus.

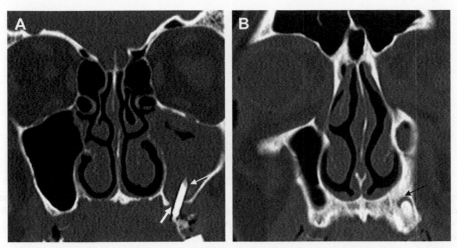

Fig. 15. Iatrogenic odontogenic sinusitis. Coronal CT image (*A*) demonstrates a displaced dental implant (*long arrow*) into the left maxillary sinus with an oroantral fistula (*short arrow*) and an opacified left maxillary sinus. The remaining sinuses are clear. In addition, note is made of periapical lucency involving one of the adjacent left maxillary teeth (*arrow* in *B*) compatible with periapical abscess.

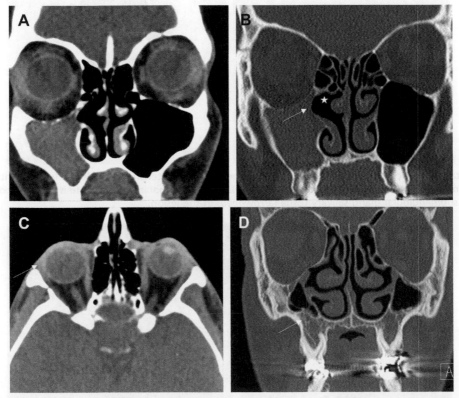

Fig. 16. Atelectatic versus hypoplastic maxillary sinus. Coronal CT images (*A*, *B*) demonstrate lateral retraction of the uncinate process (*arrow* in *B*), widening of the lateral nasal cavity (*star* in *B*), and inferior bowing of the orbital floor compatible with atelectatic maxillary sinus. This patient presented with hypoglobus (inferior displacement of the globe in the orbit), and this represented silent sinus syndrome. On the other hand, hypoplastic maxillary sinus (*C*, *D*) demonstrates enlargement of the alveolar process of the maxillary sinus (*arrow* in *D*), indicating that it did not develop normally, in contrast to silent sinus syndrome whereby the maxillary sinuses are otherwise well developed. Note that many findings on imaging may be similar between the 2 entities, including bowing of the inferior orbital wall, and lateral retraction of the uncinate process.

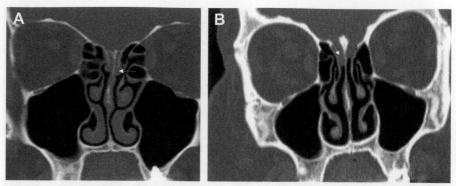

Fig. 17. Opacified olfactory cleft. Coronal CT image (*A*) demonstrates small polypoid opacities in the olfactory clefts (*arrow*). Overlying cribriform plate is intact in this patient with REAH. Contrast that with small meningoceles in the same location (*B*), characterized by dehiscence of the overlying cribriform plate (*arrow*). (Image A courtesy of Dr. Deborah Shatzkes, Lenox Hill Hospital.)

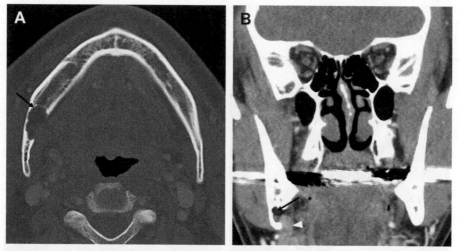

Fig. 18. Stafne bone cyst. On the axial CT image (*A*), there is a characteristic lucent lesion in the right mandible posterior margin with remodeling of the cortex (*arrow*). On the coronal image (*B*), note is made of both fat (*arrow*) and submandibular gland salivary tissue (*arrowhead*) in the lesion.

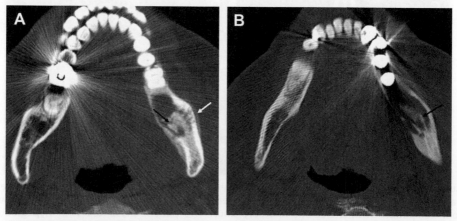

Fig. 19. Medication-related osteonecrosis of the jaw. Axial CT image (*A*) in a patient on zoledronate for metastatic breast cancer demonstrates a sclerotic lesion in the left mandible with a central sequestrum (*black arrow*) and peripheral periosteal reaction (*white arrow*). Very similar findings are seen in another patient (*B*) with actinomyces osteomyelitis of the left mandible characterized by a mandibular lucency with a central sequestrum (*arrow*). History is critical in differentiating between the entities.

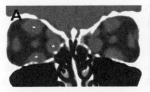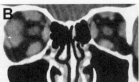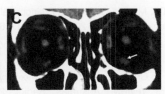

Fig. 20. Extraocular muscle enlargement. (*A*) Characteristic bilateral enlargement of the inferior rectus medial rectus and superior rectus muscles (*stars*) and increased orbital fat, compatible with thyroid orbitopathy. Contrast this with the patient in (*B*), where the muscle enlargement is unilateral and predominantly involves the lateral rectus muscle (*star*). This was the case of a pseudotumor of the orbit/idiopathic orbital inflammatory syndrome. In a patient with lipogenic variant of Graves disease (*C*), there is increased intraorbital fat; however, the extraocular muscles are not enlarged. There does appear to be hypoattenuation (*arrow*) within the muscles, which could reflect mucopolysaccharide deposition.

thyroid orbitopathy can simply present with increased intraorbital fat with the muscle being relatively normal in size (lipogenic Graves disease)[9,10] (**Fig. 20**C).

ORBITAL HEMATIC CYST

Chronic hematic cyst orbit is an orbital mass related to evolution of intraorbital hemorrhage.[11] There is an accumulation of blood products surrounded by a fibrous pseudocapsule in the chronic setting, leading to bony remodeling. This lesion may be found months to years after remote trauma to the orbit. In addition to blunt trauma, these lesions may be related to spontaneous bleeding into the orbit. On CT scan, the findings are nonspecific, hypoattenuating, or isoattenuating to soft tissue with remodeling of the adjacent bone (**Fig. 21**). On MR imaging, the lesion demonstrates increased signal on T1-weighted image and either increased or decreased signal on T2-weighted images. Imaging appearance can mimic a subperiosteal abscess or hematoma.

DISCLOSURE

The author has nothing to disclose.

CLINICS CARE POINTS

- The skull base should be scrutinized for surgical landmines on preoperative CT sinus imaging for Functional Endoscopic Sinus Surgery.
- A hyperostotic stalk is a useful imaging feature to differentiate inverted papilloma from other entities opacifying the maxillary sinus.
- MRI is useful in evaluating sinus masses to differentiate obstructed secretions from neoplasm and inflammatory disease.
- Scrutinize the images for signs of idiopathic intracranial hypertension in patients with rhinorrhea since this may represent CSF leak.
- Examine images for dental source of infection in patients with sinusitis.

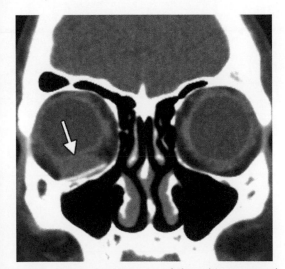

Fig. 21. Chronic hematic cyst of the orbit. A coronal CT image demonstrates a cystic lesion in the right inferior orbit displacing the globe (*arrow*). There is an adjacent silastic orbital floor implant from remote trauma. Pathology revealed chronic products compatible with hematic cyst.

REFERENCES

1. O'Brien WT Sr, Hamelin S, Weitzel EK. The preoperative sinus CT: avoiding a "CLOSE" call with surgical complications. Radiology 2016;281(1): 10–21.
2. Lee HS, Koh YC, Roh HG, et al. Secondary aneurysmal bone cyst in a craniofacial fibrous dysplasia: case report. Brain Tumor Res Treat 2018;6(2):86–91.

3. Ginat DT, Moonis G. Case 217: sinonasal organized hematoma. Radiology 2015;275(2):613–6.

4. Whyte A, Boeddinghaus R. Imaging of odontogenic sinusitis. Clin Radiol 2019;74(7):503–16.

5. Whyte A, Chapeikin G. Opaque maxillary antrum: a pictorial review. Australas Radiol 2005;49(3): 203–13.

6. Hawley KA, Ahmed M, Sindwani R. CT findings of si-nonasal respiratory epithelial adenomatoid hamar-toma: a closer look at the olfactory clefts. AJNR AmJ Neuroradiol 2013;34(5):1086–90.

7. Branstetter BF, Weissman JL, Kaplan SB. Imaging of a Stafne bone cavity: what MR adds and why a new name is needed. AJNR Am J Neuroradiol 1999; 20(4):587–9.

8. Baba A, Goto TK, Ojiri H, et al. CT imaging features of antiresorptive agent-related osteonecrosis of the jaw/medication-related osteonecrosis of the jaw. Dentomaxillofac Radiol 2018;47(4):20170323.

9. Rubin PA, Watkins LM, Rumelt S, et al. Orbital computed tomographic characteristics of globe subluxation in thyroid orbitopathy. Ophthalmology 1998;105(11):2061–4.

10. Regensburg NI, Wiersinga WM, Berendschot TT, et al. Do subtypes of Graves' orbitopathy exist? Ophthalmology 2011;118(1):191–6.

11. Iwata A, Matsumoto T, Mase M, et al. Chronic, traumatic intraconal hematic cyst of the orbit removed through the fronto-orbital approach–case report. Neurol Med Chir (Tokyo) 2000;40(2): 106–9.

Pearls and Pitfalls in Neck Imaging

Ariel Botwin, MD[a], Amy Juliano, MD[b],*

KEYWORDS

- Neck imaging • Radiology • Pearls • Pitfalls • Computed tomography
- Magnetic resonance imaging

KEY POINTS

- Interpretation of neck imaging can be challenging due to complex anatomy and pathologic entities that may share similar imaging features.
- Pitfalls in neck imaging include mistaking a normal anatomic structure for pathologic condition, mistaking anatomic asymmetry resulting from a unilateral cranial nerve palsy for a mass, identifying a lesion but committing an error of interpretation, mistaking the anatomic location of a lesion thereby generating an incorrect set of differential diagnoses, and missing a lesion because of relying on the wrong imaging modality.
- Avoiding these pitfalls improves the interpretative accuracy and positively affects patient care.

INTRODUCTION

The neck is a complex anatomic region containing multiple fascial compartments, important neural elements, and an intricate nodal drainage system. Pathologic processes in the neck can have seemingly confounding imaging appearances. Furthermore, the neck can be imaged with multiple modalities including ultrasound, computed tomography (CT), and magnetic resonance imaging (MRI). These factors render interpretation of neck imaging challenging. This article discusses several common and important pearls and pitfalls encountered in neck imaging.

MISTAKING A NORMAL ANATOMIC STRUCTURE FOR PATHOLOGY
The Thoracic Duct

The cervical portion of the thoracic duct can be identified on imaging in some cases (**Fig. 1**).[1] Familiarity with the typical anatomic location and configuration of the thoracic duct is essential for avoiding this pitfall. The cervical portion of the thoracic duct is most commonly identified at the junction between the left internal jugular and left subclavian veins.[1] It courses toward the tracheoesophageal groove and inferiorly into the thorax. In most cases, it is seen as a tubular structure.[1] At times, however, it may be more focally lobulated, mimicking a lymph node or abnormal mass such as a neurogenic tumor, although these latter entities tend to be more round in appearance.[1,2] Also, in contrast to a neurogenic tumor, the thoracic duct does not demonstrate enhancement after intravenous contrast administration.[1,2] When in doubt, an ultrasound may be performed for clarification; the thoracic duct should be easily compressible and effaced when applying pressure on the transducer.[3]

Supraclavicular Venous Varix

Occasionally, a supraclavicular venous varix may mimic an enlarged supraclavicular lymph node (**Fig. 2**). In the case of a nonenhanced CT or MRI, it can also be mistaken for an arterial aneurysm or pseudoaneurysm. Knowledge of normal venous anatomy and following the venous structures on sequential image slices should help avoid this error.[4] Coronal and sagittal reformats can be

[a] Massachusetts General Hospital, 55 Fruit Street, Boston, MA 02114, USA; [b] Massachusetts Eye and Ear, 243 Charles Street, Boston, MA 02114, USA

* Corresponding author.

E-mail address: amy_juliano@meei.harvard.edu

Neuroimag Clin N Am 32 (2022) 375–390
https://doi.org/10.1016/j.nic.2022.02.002

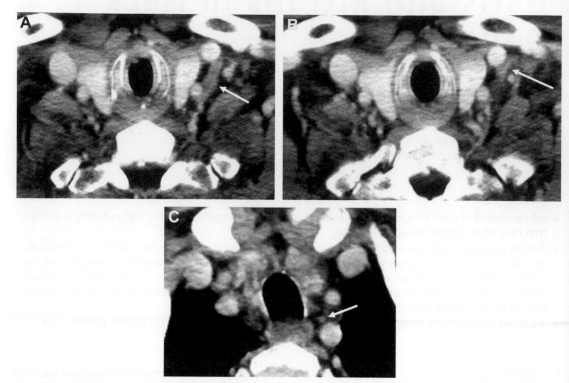

Fig. 1. Normal appearance of the cervical portion of the thoracic duct. (A) Axial contrast-enhanced CT image at the level of the thyroid gland demonstrates a soft tissue attenuation tubular structure (*arrow*) along the lateral aspect of the left internal jugular vein and left common carotid artery, corresponding to the thoracic duct. (B) Additional image more inferiorly demonstrates insertion of the thoracic duct (*arrow*) into the left internal jugular vein near the junction with the left subclavian vein. (C) An image at the level of the thoracic inlet shows the thoracic duct (*arrow*) coursing inferiorly toward the tracheoesophageal groove.

particularly helpful for following the course of venous structures in the supraclavicular region.

Posterior Belly of the Digastric Muscle

The posterior belly of the digastric muscle is located laterally in the suprahyoid neck, which is an area rich in lymph nodes. It originates from the notch of the mastoid process and courses anteroinferiorly toward the hyoid bone (Fig. 3).[5] Following the course of the muscle to the bony attachments on sequential image slices can help one distinguish it from a mass or lymph node. The sagittal reformat can be particularly helpful for visualizing the muscle origin at the mastoid process.

Asymmetry of the Anterior Bellies of the Digastric Muscle

Hypoplasia of the anterior belly of the digastric muscle is a normal anatomic variant (Fig. 4).[6,7] In contrast to denervation atrophy, no associated atrophy of the ipsilateral mylohyoid muscle would be observed.[8] Hypoplasia of the anterior belly of the digastric muscle can also result in compensatory hypertrophy of the contralateral anterior belly of the digastric muscle, which can be confused for an enlarged submental lymph node or other mass.[7] Recognizing that the hypertrophied muscle follows the same attenuation on CT and signal intensity on MRI as other muscles in the neck can help one avoid making this error.

Mylohyoid Boutonniere

Mylohyoid boutonniere refers to a congenital defect in the mylohyoid muscle and is commonly encountered on cross-sectional imaging.[9,10] Occasionally, contents of the sublingual space, including fat or the sublingual gland, can herniate through the defect and mimic a submandibular mass both clinically and radiologically.[9,10] Visualization of a focal discontinuity in the mylohyoid allows one to distinguish herniated sublingual salivary tissue from a submandibular lymph node or other soft tissue mass (Fig. 5).

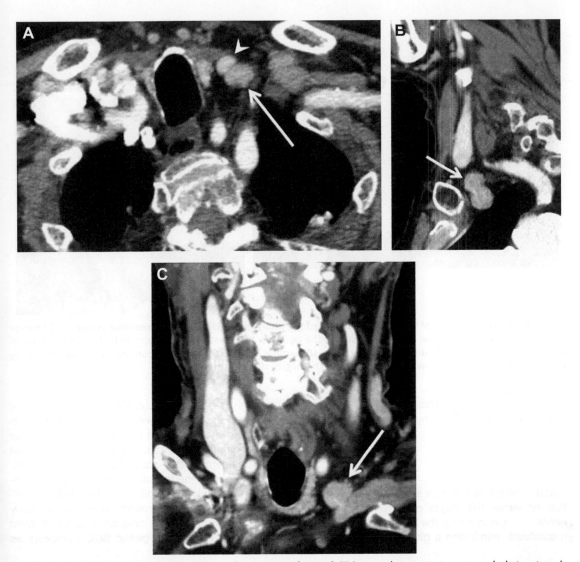

Fig. 2. Supraclavicular venous varix. (*A*) Axial contrast-enhanced CT image demonstrates a rounded structure in the left medial supraclavicular region with apparent contrast enhancement (*arrow*) adjacent to the left internal jugular vein (*arrowhead*). Sagittal (*B*) and coronal (*C*) contrast-enhanced CT images demonstrate contiguity of this structure (*arrows*) with the left subclavian vein, compatible with a supraclavicular venous varix.

MISTAKING SEQUELA OF A CRANIAL NERVE PALSY FOR A MASS
Hypoglossal Nerve Paresis

In patients with hypoglossal nerve paresis, the denervated and fatty-replaced hemitongue prolapses posteriorly into the oropharynx, masquerading as a base of tongue neoplasm (**Fig. 6**).[11,12] There are several imaging features that aid in distinguishing between these two entities. With hypoglossal nerve paresis, there is a well-defined linear zone of transition separating the signal or attenuation alteration in the denervated hemitongue from the normal contralateral hemitongue.[12] This is in contrast to a base of tongue neoplasm, which typically demonstrates an ill-defined margin with respect to the normal portion of the tongue.[12] Furthermore, with hypoglossal nerve paresis, there is preservation of some normal tongue muscle striations, which may be obliterated by a base of tongue neoplasm.[12] Acutely, the denervated hemitongue demonstrates diffusely increased T2 signal on MRI, reflecting denervation edema.[11] In the chronic setting, the affected hemitongue undergoes fatty atrophy, which can be appreciated on CT as fat attenuation and on MRI as T1-hyperintense signal.[11] Finally, when suspecting a

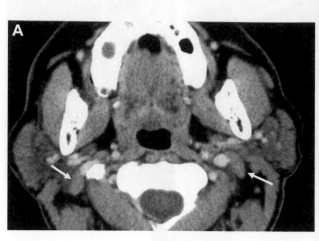

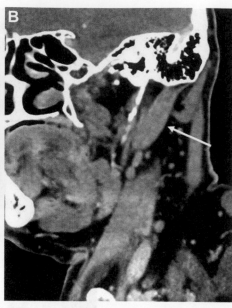

Fig. 3. Normal appearance of the posterior bellies of the digastric muscles. (*A*) Axial contrast-enhanced CT image at the level of the mandibular rami demonstrates the posterior bellies of the digastric muscles bilaterally (*arrows*) as they pass adjacent to the internal jugular veins. (*B*) Sagittal oblique CT image demonstrates the posterior belly of the digastric muscle (*arrow*) originating from the notch of the mastoid process.

hypoglossal nerve paresis, a thorough search along the course of the hypoglossal nerve may reveal a causative lesion.

Vocal Cord Paresis

Vocal cord paresis occurs secondary to dysfunction of either the vagus or recurrent laryngeal nerve.[13,14] On imaging, the affected vocal cord is medialized, mimicking a glottic lesion such as a squamous cell carcinoma (SCC; **Fig. 7**).[13] Other features associated with vocal cord paresis include dilatation of the ipsilateral pyriform sinus and laryngeal ventricle, thickening and medial displacement of the ipsilateral aryepiglottic fold, and atrophy of the ipsilateral posterior cricoarytenoid muscle when chronic.[13,15] When this constellation of findings is present, one can be fairly confident in making a diagnosis of vocal cord paresis. In contrast, a glottic SCC manifests as

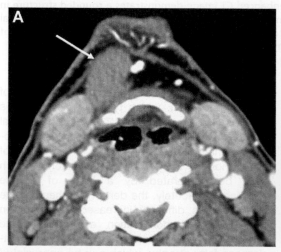

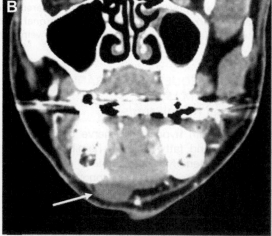

Fig. 4. Asymmetry of the anterior bellies of the digastric muscles. Axial (*A*) and coronal (*B*) contrast-enhanced CT images show absence of the anterior belly of the left digastric muscle and compensatory hypertrophy of the anterior belly of the right digastric muscle (*arrows*).

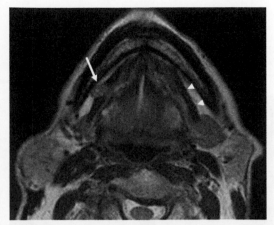

Fig. 5. Right mylohyoid boutonniere. Axial T2-weighted image at the level of the floor of mouth demonstrates a focal defect in the right mylohyoid through which the sublingual gland (*white arrow*) herniates into the submandibular space. Note the left mylohyoid (white *arrowheads*) without any focal defects.

enhancing asymmetric soft tissue thickening involving the true vocal cord.[13,14] Furthermore, extension to the adjacent laryngeal cartilages with asymmetric sclerosis or frank erosion raises the suspicion for a glottic malignancy.[13]

IDENTIFYING A LESION BUT COMMITTING AN ERROR OF INTERPRETATION
Paraganglioma Versus Schwannoma

Vagal paragangliomas and schwannomas both arise along the course of the vagus nerve, located between the carotid artery and internal jugular vein within the poststyloid parapharyngeal space (also referred to as the carotid space), and both demonstrate enhancement after intravenous contrast administration.[16] However, a paraganglioma can be distinguished from a schwannoma based on its characteristic MRI appearance of multiple intratumoral flow voids, classically termed the "salt and pepper" appearance (**Figs. 8** and **9**).[16–18] Also of note, paragangliomas cause destructive/permeative bony change, whereas schwannomas cause smooth adjacent bony remodeling.[16] This feature can be helpful for distinguishing paraganglioma from schwannoma when these tumors are located within the jugular foramen. When large, schwannomas may contain cystic components, a feature not generally seen with paragangliomas.[16] Finally, paragangliomas demonstrate uptake on Gallium-68 DOTATATE positron emission tomography (PET), which is considered a first line nuclear medicine imaging modality for detection of these tumors.[19]

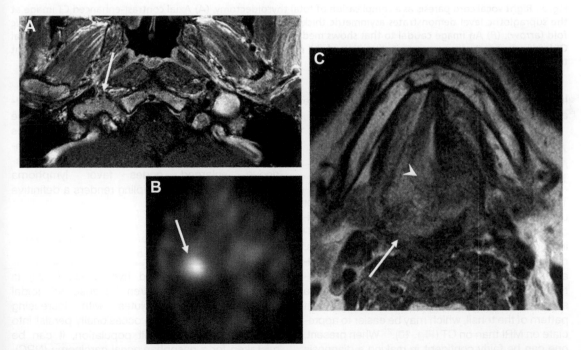

Fig. 6. Right hypoglossal nerve paresis secondary to a glomus jugulare paraganglioma. (*A*) Axial postcontrast T1-weighted image through the skull base demonstrates an enhancing lesion (*arrow*) extending from the right jugular foramen to the right hypoglossal canal. (*B*) Axial Octreotide single photon emission computed tomography image demonstrates intense radiotracer uptake within the lesion (*arrow*), compatible with a glomus jugulare paraganglioma. (*C*) Axial T1-weighted image depicts posterior protrusion (*arrow*) and fatty replacement (*arrowhead*) of the right hemitongue musculature.

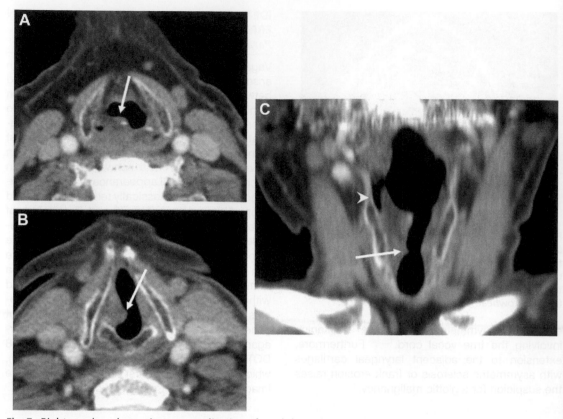

Fig. 7. Right vocal cord paresis as a complication of total thyroidectomy. (*A*) Axial contrast-enhanced CT image at the supraglottic level demonstrates asymmetric thickening and medial displacement of the right aryepiglottic fold (*arrow*). (*B*) An image caudal to that shows medialization of the true right vocal cord (*arrow*). (*C*) Coronal CT image demonstrates asymmetric dilatation of the right pyriform sinus (*arrowhead*) and thinning of the right true vocal cord (*arrow*) as compared with the left.

In contrast, schwannomas do not demonstrate avidity for this radiotracer.

Tonsillitis, Squamous Cell Carcinoma, and Non-Hodgkin Lymphoma of the Palatine Tonsil

Tonsillitis typically presents as either bilateral or unilateral tonsillar enlargement with reactive cervical lymphadenopathy.[20] This constellation of findings can be confused for a neoplastic process, mainly non-Hodgkin lymphoma or SCC of the palatine tonsil with metastatic adenopathy. A relatively specific imaging finding for tonsillitis is a striated appearance and striated enhancement pattern of the tonsil, which may be easier to appreciate on MRI than on CT (**Fig. 10**).[20] When present, one can be fairly confident in making a diagnosis of tonsillitis. If not present, short-term clinical and possibly imaging follow-up may be necessary for confirmation. Non-Hodgkin lymphoma and SCC of the palatine tonsil can manifest similarly on imaging, both appearing as bulky tonsillar

enlargement, although unilateral involvement, heterogeneous attenuation/enhancement, and the presence of necrotic cervical nodal metastases favor the diagnosis of SCC, whereas bilateral homogeneous tonsillar enlargement and homogeneous enlarged nodes favor lymphoma (**Fig. 11**).[21,22] Tissue sampling renders a definitive diagnosis.

Nasopharyngeal Adenoid Hyperplasia Versus Nasopharyngeal Carcinoma

Nasopharyngeal adenoid hyperplasia (NAH) is most common in children because adenoidal lymphatic tissue involutes with increasing age.[23,24] However, it can occasionally persist into adulthood.[24] In the adult population, it can be mistaken for a nasopharyngeal carcinoma (NPC). In its early stage, NPC generally manifests as asymmetric soft tissue fullness in the nasopharynx, as it most commonly arises from the fossa of Rosenmüller (**Fig. 12**).[25] In its later stage, NPC can infiltrate into the adjacent deep neck

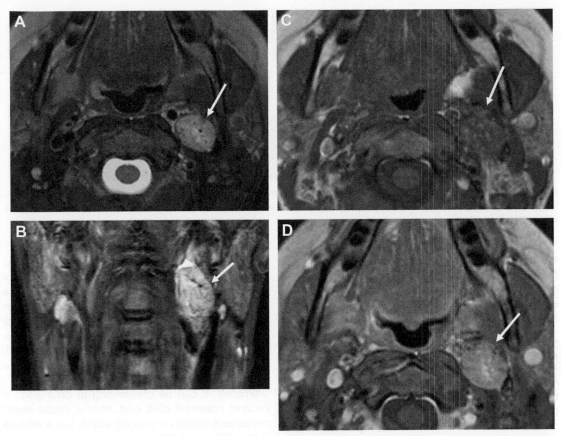

Fig. 8. Vagal paraganglioma (glomus vagale). Axial (*A*) and coronal (*B*) fat-suppressed T2-weighted images demonstrate a T2-hyperintense mass (*arrow*) containing several flow voids interposed between the left ICA and left internal jugular vein. Axial precontrast T1-weighted (*C*) and axial postcontrast fat-suppressed T1-weighted (*D*) images show that the mass (*arrows*) enhances avidly.

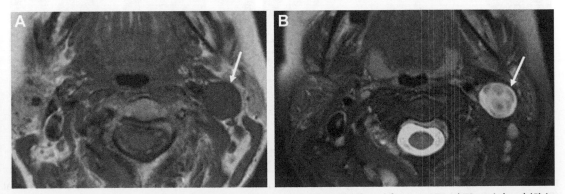

Fig. 9. Vagal schwannoma. Axial noncontrast-enhanced T1-weighted (*A*) and fat-suppressed T2-weighted (*B*) images demonstrate a T1-isointense and T2-hyperintense mass (*arrows*) situated between the left ICA and left internal jugular vein. Note the absence of flow voids within the mass.

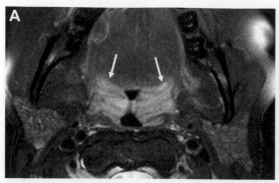
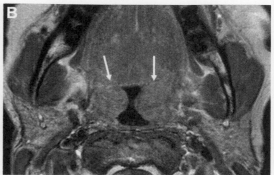

Fig. 10. Tonsillitis in a patient presenting with sore throat. Axial T2-weighted (*A*) and contrast-enhanced T1-weighted (*B*) images demonstrate enlargement and a striated appearance and enhancement pattern of the palatine tonsils (*arrows*).

spaces, skull base, and intracranial compartment.[25] In contrast to NPC, NAH manifests as symmetric soft tissue thickening with a striated enhancement pattern (**Fig. 13**).[24,26] Furthermore, NAH may contain internal retention cysts.[24,27]

Second Branchial Cleft Cyst Versus Cervical Nodal Metastasis

A second branchial cleft cyst is the most common type of branchial cleft cyst.[28] It is most often interposed between the submandibular gland and sternocleidomastoid muscle. On imaging, it typically appears as a cystic mass with a thin nonenhancing wall and demonstrates internal homogeneity.[28,29] A cystic lymph node metastasis from SCC or papillary thyroid carcinoma is more likely to demonstrate complex features, such as internal septations or mural soft tissue, heterogeneity, and a thick irregular enhancing wall in the former,

and hyperenhancing soft tissue components and calcifications in the latter.[29,30] Nonetheless, not all cystic nodal metastases demonstrate these complex imaging features; in particular, human papillomavirus (HPV)-associated oropharyngeal carcinoma often produces large cystic nodes (**Fig. 14**).[29] Furthermore, if infected or inflamed, second branchial cleft cysts can also demonstrate internal complexity and thick enhancing walls.[28,29] Ultimately, it can be challenging to distinguish a second branchial cleft cyst from a cystic nodal metastasis based on imaging alone. Other entities in the differential diagnosis include lymphatic malformation and nodal infection by Mycobacterium avium intracellulare.[28,31] Therefore, one should have a low threshold for recommending tissue sampling when encountering a cystic mass in the lateral neck, especially when the lesion is seen in an adult patient.

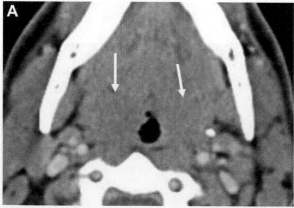
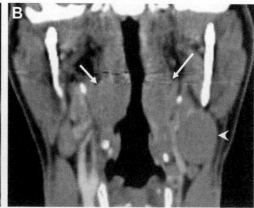

Fig. 11. Non-Hodgkin lymphoma involving the palatine tonsils and cervical lymph nodes. Axial (*A*) and coronal (*B*) contrast-enhanced CT images demonstrate prominence of the bilateral palatine tonsils (*arrows*). An enlarged nonnecrotic left level IIA lymph node (*arrowhead*) is seen on the coronal image. Note the homogeneous attenuation of the palatine tonsils and the lack of a striated enhancement pattern.

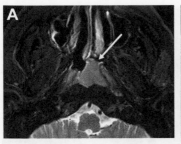
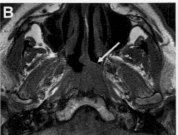
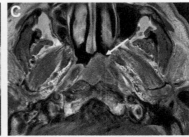

Fig. 12. NPC. Axial fat-suppressed T2-weighted (*A*), precontrast T1-weighted (*B*), and postcontrast T1-weighted (*C*) images demonstrate asymmetric enhancing soft tissue (*arrows*) centered in the left aspect of the nasopharynx crossing midline and protruding anteriorly toward the left nasal choana. Note that the fossae of Rosenmüller are effaced.

Laryngeal Saccular Cyst Versus Laryngeal Mass

A laryngeal saccular cyst is defined as a fluid-filled dilatation of the laryngeal appendix, which is a normal anatomic extension directed superolaterally from the ventricular apex and located between the false vocal cord and thyroid cartilage.[32] On CT, laryngeal saccular cysts are generally well-circumscribed with an imperceptible wall and demonstrate fluid attenuation (**Fig. 15**).[28,33] When these features are present, one can be fairly confident of the diagnosis of saccular cyst. However, if the cyst contains proteinaceous or hemorrhagic content, an MRI may be needed for more definitive characterization and to show no internal enhancement.[28] When the space is dilated, but is air-filled rather than fluid-filled, it is termed a laryngocele.[28] It is important to note that a saccular cyst or a laryngocele can arise secondary to a mass obstructing the ventricle.[28,32] Therefore, one should carefully examine the larynx for a glottic mass whenever a saccular cyst or laryngocele is visualized.

MISTAKING THE ANATOMIC LOCATION OF A LESION
Sympathetic Chain Schwannoma Versus Vagal Schwannoma

In most cases, a sympathetic chain schwannoma can be differentiated from a vagal nerve schwannoma based on the relationship of the mass to the adjacent vasculature. The sympathetic chain is located posteromedial to the carotid sheath and thus a sympathetic chain schwannoma typically causes anterior or anterolateral displacement of the internal carotid artery (ICA) (**Fig. 16**).[17,34] In contrast, the vagus nerve courses lateral to the ICA, between the ICA and internal jugular vein, and thus a vagal nerve schwannoma tends to splay these two vessels and displaces the ICA medially (see **Fig. 9**).[34]

Carotid Body Tumor Versus Glomus Vagale

Carotid body and glomus vagale tumors are types of paragangliomas, named for their location of origin.[16] In most cases, they can be distinguished

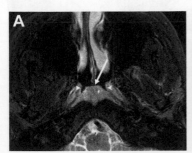
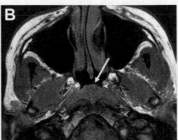
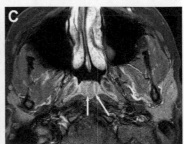

Fig. 13. NAH. Axial fat-suppressed T2-weighted (*A*) and precontrast T1-weighted (*B*) images at the level of the nasopharynx show symmetric soft tissue thickening in the nasopharynx (*arrows*) with preservation of the fossae of Rosenmüller (*arrowheads*). (*C*) Axial contrast-enhanced fat-suppressed T1-weighted image demonstrates a striated enhancement pattern of the soft tissue with multiple thin linear enhancing striations (*arrows*).

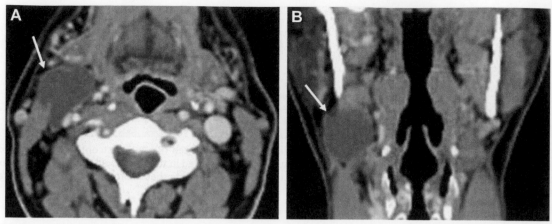

Fig. 14. Necrotic right level IIA nodal metastasis from HPV-associated tonsillar SCC. Axial (*A*) and coronal (*B*) contrast-enhanced CT images demonstrate a thin-walled cystic lesion (*arrows*) in the right lateral neck interposed between the submandibular gland and sternocleidomastoid muscle. The lesion has no discernible enhancing component and resembles a second branchial cleft cyst.

from one another based on the location from which they arise. Carotid body tumors are situated at the carotid bifurcation and splay the ICA and external carotid artery (ECA).[35] In contrast, glomus vagale tumors are typically located posterior to the carotid bifurcation.[36] However, glomus vagale tumors can also occasionally splay the ICA and ECA, posing a diagnostic challenge.[17] In these scenarios, a glomus vagale can be differentiated from a carotid body tumor by vessel encasement. A glomus vagale usually does not encase the ICA and ECA, whereas a carotid body tumor typically fills the groove of the carotid bifurcation and surrounds the ICA and ECA (ie, greater than 180° of contact with the vessels) (**Fig. 17**).[17]

Prestyloid versus Poststyloid Parapharyngeal Space Mass

The parapharyngeal space is divided into prestyloid and poststyloid compartments by the tensor styloid fascia.[37,38] The prestyloid parapharyngeal space is also simply referred to as the parapharyngeal space, and the poststyloid parapharyngeal space is also referred to as the carotid space. Masses arising in the prestyloid compartment tend to displace the carotid sheath structures posteriorly and flatten the longus muscle from anteriorly when large (**Fig. 18**), whereas masses arising in the poststyloid compartment tend to displace the carotid sheath structures anteromedially and

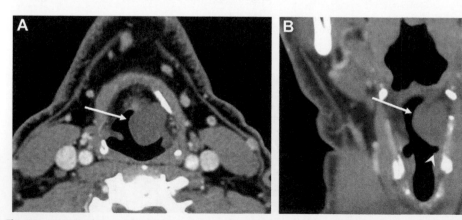

Fig. 15. Laryngeal saccular cyst. (*A*) Axial contrast-enhanced CT image shows a well-circumscribed low attenuation lesion (*arrow*) centered in the left paraglottic fat. (*B*) Coronal contrast-enhanced CT image shows that the lesion (*arrow*) bulges the left false vocal cord smoothly. There is no mass obstructing the opening of the left laryngeal ventricle (*arrowhead*).

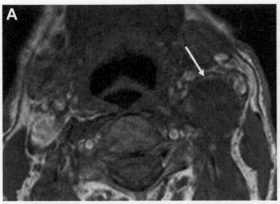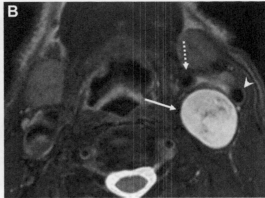

Fig. 16. Sympathetic chain schwannoma. Axial T1-weighted (*A*) and fat-suppressed T2-weighted (*B*) images demonstrate a T1-isointense and T2-hyperintense mass (*arrow*) in the left neck causing anterolateral displacement of the left ICA (*arrowhead* in *B*). The more medial flow void anterior to the lesion is the ECA (*dotted arrow* in *B*).

are lateral to the longus (see **Fig. 8**).[37] The main differential diagnosis of a prestyloid parapharyngeal space mass is a lesion related to the deep lobe of the parotid gland, most often a primary parotid neoplasm such as a pleomorphic adenoma (benign mixed tumor). The main differential diagnosis of a poststyloid parapharyngeal space mass is a paraganglioma or a neurogenic tumor such as a schwannoma.[37] Distinguishing a prestyloid from a poststyloid parapharyngeal space mass is important for the proper planning of surgical approach.[37,38]

Supraglottic Versus Hypopharyngeal Lesion

The hypopharynx contains the posterior surface of the aryepiglottic folds, pyriform sinuses, posterior hypopharyngeal wall, and postcricoid region.[39,40] It is bounded superiorly by the pharyngoepiglottic folds and inferiorly by the pharyngoesophageal junction. In contrast, the supraglottis is located more anteriorly and contains the anterior surface of the aryepiglottic folds, paraglottic fat, arytenoids, and false vocal cords. It is bounded superiorly by the epiglottis and inferiorly by the superior surface of the true vocal cords. Recognizing the distinction between these two anatomic compartments is essential for classification and staging of tumors that arise in this region (**Fig. 19**).[40]

MISSING PATHOLOGY AS A CONSEQUENCE OF RELYING ON THE WRONG IMAGING MODALITY
Thyroid Nodules on CT

Ultrasound is the gold standard imaging modality for detection and characterization of thyroid nodules.[41] To date, studies have found no reliable features specific to a nodule itself on CT that can distinguish a benign from potentially malignant thyroid nodule; most indicators are related to associated findings (eg, the presence of abnormal nodes suspicious for metastatic disease), patient demographic (eg, pediatric population), or findings on another imaging modality (eg, increased fluorodeoxyglucose [FDG] avidity on PET).[41] Furthermore, thyroid nodules can be missed on CT not only due to inherent contrast limitation but also as a result of streak artifact from the adjacent clavicles or high density intravenous contrast in the subclavian veins (**Fig. 20**).[42] As such, one should use caution when stating that the thyroid gland has a normal appearance solely by CT.

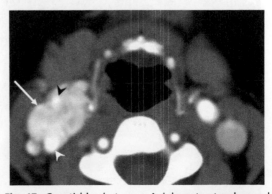

Fig. 17. Carotid body tumor. Axial contrast-enhanced CT image at the level of the hyoid bone demonstrates an avidly enhancing mass (*arrow*) centered in the right carotid bifurcation. It splays and encases the right internal (*white arrowhead*) and external (*black arrowhead*) carotid arteries.

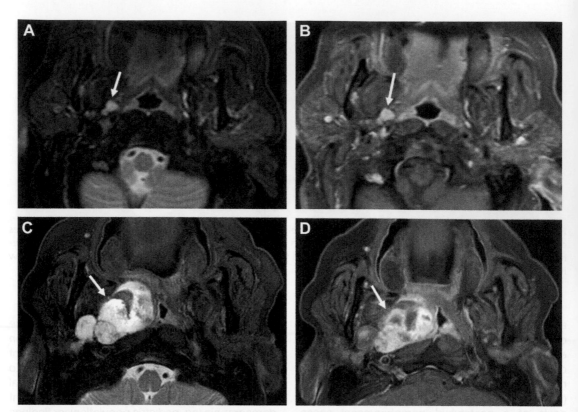

Fig. 18. Pleomorphic adenoma arising from the deep lobe parotid in the prestyloid parapharyngeal space. Fat-suppressed T2-weighted (*A*) and contrast-enhanced fat-suppressed T1-weighted (*B*) images demonstrate a T2-hyperintense homogenously enhancing mass (*arrows*) in the right prestyloid parapharyngeal space. Thirteen years later, repeat imaging (*C* and *D*), same pulse sequences as *A* and *B*, respectively, showed substantial interval growth of the mass (*arrows*), now displacing the pharyngeal wall medially and flattening the longus muscle posteriorly, and appearing heterogeneous. This represented progression of a recurrent pleomorphic adenoma; the original tumor was excised 5 years before the first scan shown in *A* and *B*.

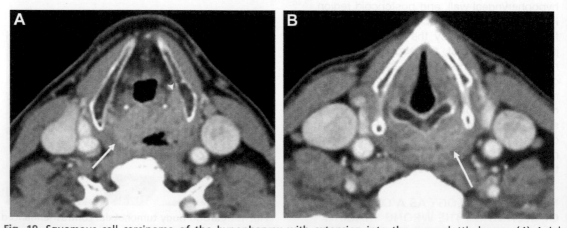

Fig. 19. Squamous cell carcinoma of the hypopharynx with extension into the supraglottic larynx. (*A*) Axial contrast-enhanced CT image demonstrates ill-defined enhancing soft tissue involving the posterior hypopharyngeal wall (*arrow*) extending into the left supraglottic paraglottic fat of the larynx (*arrowhead*). (*B*) Additional axial contrast-enhanced CT image caudal to that demonstrates ill-defined enhancing soft tissue (*arrow*) involving the postcricoid region of the hypopharynx.

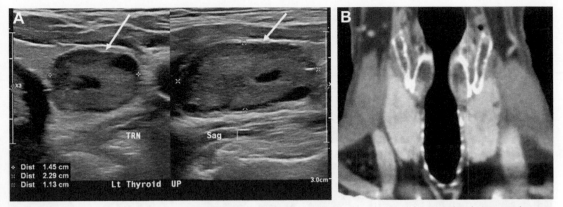

Fig. 20. Thyroid nodule detected on ultrasound but not CT. (*A*) Transverse and longitudinal gray-scale sonographic images demonstrate a predominantly solid nodule with cystic components measuring up to 2.3 cm (*arrow*) in the upper pole of the left thyroid lobe. (*B*) On subsequent contrast-enhanced neck CT obtained for preoperative planning, the nodule is essentially not visualized. The nodule was found to represent a Hurthle cell adenoma on surgical pathology.

Paranasal Sinus Disease on MRI

Occasionally paranasal sinus disease can be mistakenly interpreted as normal sinus aeration on MRI (**Fig. 21**).[43,44] This is because highly proteinaceous secretions or secretions colonized by fungus can cause extremely hypointense signal or signal dropout, akin to air.[44] Therefore, CT should serve as a first line imaging modality for paranasal sinus disease evaluation, with MRI reserved for lesion characterization.

Salivary Gland Masses on CT

Salivary gland masses can have similar Hounsfield attenuation to normal gland parenchyma, rendering them difficult to detect by CT.[45] This is less of a concern with MRI, which demonstrates superior soft tissue contrast as compared with CT and is not density dependent (**Fig. 22**).[45,46] However, enhancing tumors are sometimes less conspicuous on the postcontrast T1-weighted sequences than the other sequences by blending in

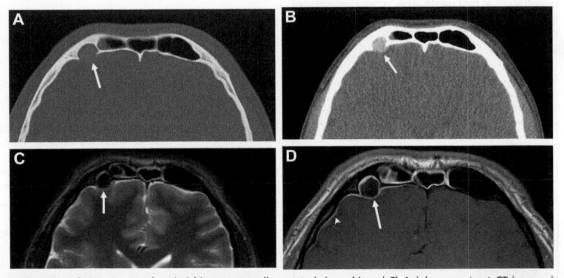

Fig. 21. Frontal sinus mucocele mimicking a normally aerated sinus. (*A* and *B*) Axial noncontrast CT images in bone and soft tissue algorithms at the level of the frontal sinuses demonstrate hyperattenuating material in a right frontal sinus air cell with associated dehiscence of the frontal sinus inner table, compatible with a mucocele (*arrows*). (*C* and *D*) Axial T2-weighted and contrast-enhanced T1-weighted images at the same level demonstrate hypointense signal within the mucocele, mimicking an aerated air cell (*arrow*). Note that there is mild thin enhancement of the dura overlying the right frontal convexity (*arrow* in D). This is likely reactive to the underlying mucocele.

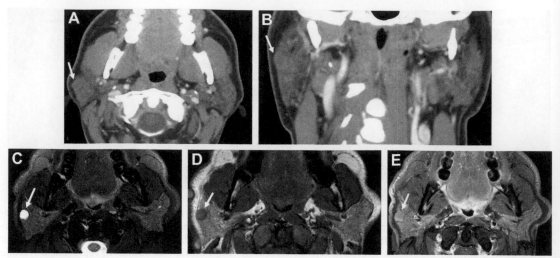

Fig. 22. Parotid gland lesion more conspicuous on MRI. Axial (*A*) and coronal (*B*) contrast-enhanced CT images show a subtle lesion in the superficial right parotid gland (*arrows*) reflecting a parotid nodule, which is nearly isoattenuating relative to the normal parotid gland parenchyma and can be easily missed. Axial T2-weighted (*C*), precontrast T1-weighted (*D*), and postcontrast fat-suppressed T1-weighted (*D*) images clearly demonstrate the nodule as a well-circumscribed T2-hyperintense and T1-hypointense lesion (*arrow*) in the superficial right parotid gland, corresponding to the finding seen on CT. Note that the lesion is also more conspicuous on the noncontrast T1 and T2-weighted sequences than on the postcontrast T1-weighted sequence. Fine needle aspiration of this nodule was nondiagnostic and demonstrated crystals and proteinaceous debris. The patient opted for close imaging follow-up of this nodule.

with the normal parotid tissue, leading to the so-called disappearing tumor phenomenon. Ultrasound is also a better alternative to CT for detection of salivary gland masses if the lesion is superficial enough and amenable to sound wave penetration at that depth. This is because salivary gland masses tend to be hypoechoic relative to the normal hyperechoic nature of normal gland parenchyma.[45]

CLINICS CARE POINTS

- Normal anatomic structures in the neck can be mistaken for pathology.

- Cranial nerve palsies that can result in imaging findings mimicking masses include hypoglossal nerve and vocal cord paresis.

- Some lesions in the neck are challenging to distinguish from one another due to their similarity in location and imaging appearance.

- Mistaking the anatomic location of a neck lesion may lead to an erroneous differential diagnosis.

- Reliance on the correct imaging modality is pivotal for detecting neck pathology.

DISCLOSURE

The authors have neither a funding source nor financial or commercial conflicts of interest to disclose.

REFERENCES

1. Liu ME, Branstetter BF, Whetstone J, et al. Normal CT appearance of the distal thoracic duct. AJR Am J Roentgenol 2006;187(6):1615–20.

2. Kami YN, Chikui T, Okamura K, et al. Imaging findings of neurogenic tumours in the head and neck region. Dentomaxillofac Radiol 2012;41(1):18–23.

3. Seeger M, Bewig B, Günther R, et al. Terminal part of thoracic duct: high-resolution US imaging. Radiology 2009;252(3):897–904.

4. Escott EJ, Branstetter BF. It's not a cervical lymph node, it's a vein: CT and MR imaging findings in the veins of the head and neck. Radiographics 2006;26(5):1501–15.

5. Kim SD, Loukas M. Anatomy and variations of digastric muscle. Anat Cell Biol 2019;52(1):1–11.

6. Aktekin M, Kurtoğlu Z, Oztürk AH. A bilateral and symmetrical variation of the anterior belly of the digastric muscle. Acta Med Okayama 2003;57(4):205–7.

7. Ochoa-Escudero M, Juliano AF. Unilateral hypoplasia with contralateral hypertrophy of anterior belly of digastric muscle: a case report. Surg Radiol Anat 2016;38(8):973–4.

8. Russo CP, Smoker WR, Weissman JL. MR appearance of trigeminal and hypoglossal motor denervation. AJNR Am J Neuroradiol 1997;18(7):1375–83.

9. Patel S, Bhatt AA. Imaging of the sublingual and submandibular spaces. Insights Imaging 2018; 9(3):391–401.

10. La'porte SJ, Juttla JK, Lingam RK. Imaging the floor of the mouth and the sublingual space. Radiographics 2011;31(5):1215–30.

11. Law CP, Chandra RV, Hoang JK, et al. Imaging the oral cavity: key concepts for the radiologist. Br J Radiol 2011;84(1006):944–57.

12. Learned KO, Thaler ER, O'Malley BW Jr, et al. Hypoglossal nerve palsy missed and misinterpreted: the hidden skull base. J Comput Assist Tomogr 2012; 36(6):718–24.

13. Paquette CM, Manos DC, Psooy BJ. Unilateral vocal cord paralysis: a review of CT findings, mediastinal causes, and the course of the recurrent laryngeal nerves. Radiographics 2012;32(3):721–40.

14. Dankbaar JW, Pameijer FA. Vocal cord paralysis: anatomy, imaging and pathology. Insights into imaging 2014;5(6):743–51.

15. Chin SC, Edelstein S, Chen CY, et al. Using CT to localize side and level of vocal cord paralysis. AJR Am J Roentgenol 2003;180(4):1165–70.

16. Rao AB, Koeller KK, Adair CF. From the archives of the AFIP. Paragangliomas of the head and neck: radiologic-pathologic correlation. Armed Forces Institute of Pathology. Radiographics 1999;19(6): 1605–32.

17. Anil G, Tan TY. Imaging characteristics of schwannoma of the cervical sympathetic chain: a review of 12 cases. AJNR Am J Neuroradiol 2010;31(8):1408–12.

18. Olsen WL, Dillon WP, Kelly WM, et al. MR imaging of paragangliomas. AJR Am J Roentgenol 1987; 148(1):201–4.

19. Chang CA, Pattison DA, Tothill RW, et al. 68)Ga-DOTATATE and (18)F-FDG PET/CT in paraganglioma and pheochromocytoma: utility, patterns and heterogeneity. Cancer Imaging 2016;16(1):22.

20. Capps EF, Kinsella JJ, Gupta M, et al. Emergency imaging assessment of acute, nontraumatic conditions of the head and neck. Radiographics 2010; 30(5):1335–52.

21. Urquhart AC, Hutchins LG, Berg RL. Distinguishing non-Hodgkin lymphoma from squamous cell carcinoma tumors of the head and neck by computed tomography parameters. Laryngoscope 2002;112(6): 1079–83.

22. Wang XY, Wu N, Zhu Z, et al. Computed tomography features of enlarged tonsils as a first symptom of non-Hodgkin's lymphoma. Chin J Cancer 2010; 29(5):556–60.

23. Vogler RC, Ii FJ, Pilgram TK. Age-specific size of the normal adenoid pad on magnetic resonance imaging. Clin Otolaryngol Allied Sci 2000;25(5):392–5.

24. Surov A, Ryl I, Bartel-Friedrich S, et al. MRI of nasopharyngeal adenoid hypertrophy. Neuroradiol J 2016;29(5):408–12.

25. Hoe J. CT of nasopharyngeal carcinoma: significance of widening of the preoccipital soft tissue on axial scans. AJR Am J Roentgenol 1989;153(4):867–72.

26. King AD, Vlantis AC, Bhatia KS, et al. Primary nasopharyngeal carcinoma: diagnostic accuracy of MR imaging versus that of endoscopy and endoscopic biopsy. Radiology 2011;258(2):531–7.

27. Bhatia KS, King AD, Vlantis AC, et al. Nasopharyngeal mucosa and adenoids: appearance at MR imaging. Radiology 2012;263(2):437–43.

28. Koeller KK, Alamo L, Adair CF, et al. Congenital cystic masses of the neck: radiologic-pathologic correlation. Radiographics 1999;19(1):121–46. quiz 152-123.

29. Goyal N, Zacharia TT, Goldenberg D. Differentiation of branchial cleft cysts and malignant cystic adenopathy of pharyngeal origin. AJR Am J Roentgenol 2012;199(2):W216–21.

30. Hoang JK, Lee WK, Lee M, et al. US Features of thyroid malignancy: pearls and pitfalls. Radiographics 2007;27(3):847–60 [discussion 861-845].

31. Robson CD, Hazra R, Barnes PD, et al. Nontuberculous mycobacterial infection of the head and neck in immunocompetent children: CT and MR findings. AJNR Am J Neuroradiol 1999;20(10):1829–35.

32. Young VN, Smith LJ. Saccular cysts: a current review of characteristics and management. Laryngoscope 2012;122(3):595–9.

33. Glazer HS, Mauro MA, Aronberg DJ, et al. Computed tomography of laryngoceles. AJR Am J Roentgenol 1983;140(3):549–52.

34. Furukawa M, Furukawa MK, Katoh K, et al. Differentiation between schwannoma of the vagus nerve and schwannoma of the cervical sympathetic chain by imaging diagnosis. Laryngoscope 1996;106(12 Pt 1):1548–52.

35. Hoang VT, Trinh CT, Lai TAK, et al. Carotid body tumor: a case report and literature review. J Radiol Case Rep 2019;13(8):19–30.

36. Chengazi HU, Bhatt AA. Pathology of the carotid space. Insights into imaging 2019;10(1):21.

37. Shin JH, Lee HK, Kim SY, et al. Imaging of parapharyngeal space lesions: focus on the prestyloid compartment. AJR Am J Roentgenol 2001;177(6):1465–70.

38. Zhi K, Ren W, Zhou H, et al. Management of parapharyngeal-space tumors. J Oral Maxillofac Surg 2009;67(6):1239–44.

39. Tao TY, Menias CO, Herman TE, et al. Easier to swallow: pictorial review of structural findings of the pharynx at barium pharyngography. Radiographics 2013;33(7):e189–208.

40. Gupta A, Young RJ. Supraglottic larynx and hypopharynx: an important anatomic distinction. Radiographics 2011;31(1):116.

41. Grady AT, Sosa JA, Tanpitukpongse TP, et al. Radiology reports for incidental thyroid nodules on CT and MRI: high variability across subspecialties. AJNR Am J Neuroradiol 2015;36(2):397–402.

42. Ahmed S, Horton KM, Jeffrey RB Jr, et al. Incidental thyroid nodules on chest CT: review of the literature and management suggestions. AJR Am J Roentgenol 2010;195(5):1066–71.

43. Aribandi M, McCoy VA, Bazan C 3rd. Imaging features of invasive and noninvasive fungal sinusitis: a review. Radiographics 2007;27(5):1283–96.

44. Dillon WP, Som PM, Fullerton GD. Hypointense MR signal in chronically inspissated sinonasal secretions. Radiology 1990;174(1):73–8.

45. Kei PL, Tan TY. CT "invisible" lesion of the major salivary glands a diagnostic pitfall of contrast-enhanced CT. Clin Radiol 2009;64(7):744–6.

46. Christe A, Waldherr C, Hallett R, et al. MR imaging of parotid tumors: typical lesion characteristics in MR imaging improve discrimination between benign and malignant disease. AJNR Am J Neuroradiol 2011;32(7):1202–7.

Normal Vascular Structures and Variants on Head and Neck Imaging

June Kim, MD*, Edward J. Escott, MD

KEYWORDS

• Head and neck • Vascular anatomy • Variants

KEY POINTS

- Main arterial pathways from the neck to the brain are carotid and vertebral arteries.
- Two main venous pathways draining blood from the head and neck include the jugular and vertebral venous systems.
- Knowledge of variant anatomy may help with imaging diagnosis, planning for procedures, and avoiding potential complications.

INTRODUCTION

Within the neck, much attention in cross-sectional imaging is paid to learning the intricacies of mucosal structures, such as the pharynx and larynx or the anatomy of the spine. Knowledge of the normal appearances of vascular structures in the neck, however, is important in the evaluation of not only dedicated vascular studies, but also when imaging other structures. The main arteries of the neck are the carotid and vertebral systems, which supply the cerebrovascular system and structures in the neck. Venous drainage of the cerebrovascular system traverses through the neck to the chest via the jugular veins, which also collect venous drainage of neck, face, and spinal structures, and the vertebral venous system. This article discusses normal anatomy of arteries and veins of the neck and some of the skull base, and a few related structures, such as the thoracic duct. Then a selection of anatomic variants, some of which are pitfalls for image interpretation, are described.

NORMAL VASCULAR ANATOMY
Arteries

The cervical carotid arteries are comprised of the common carotid arteries (CCAs), which then bifurcate into the internal carotid arteries (ICAs), which continue intracranially to supply the intracranial anterior circulation; and external carotid arteries (ECAs), which predominantly provide branches to supply the neck and face. In the neck, each set of carotid arteries, specifically the CCA, ICA, and portions of the ECA, are wrapped within a carotid sheath, along with the internal jugular vein (IJV) and vagus nerve (**Fig. 1**).[1] In the suprahyoid neck, additional nerves, such as cranial nerves 9, 11, and 12, and lymph nodes are found within the carotid sheath.[2]

Common carotid arteries

In the upper chest, the right CCA originates as the first branch of the brachiocephalic artery (innominate artery), which is the first branch vessel of the aortic arch (**Fig. 2**).

The left CCA extends directly from a left-sided aortic arch as the next branch distal to the brachiocephalic artery (see **Fig. 2**). Sometimes, instead, the left CCA shares a common trunk with the brachiocephalic artery or the left CCA branches from the brachiocephalic artery itself. This is the most common branch pattern variant of the aorta and is seen with fair frequency.[3] This variant configuration is sometimes referred to as a "bovine arch," although "bovine" is a misnomer, because the aortic arch of a cow has a different configuration.[4]

Department of Radiology, University of Kentucky, 800 Rose Street, Lexington, KY 40536, USA
* Corresponding author.
E-mail address: june.kim@uky.edu

Neuroimag Clin N Am 32 (2022) 391–412
https://doi.org/10.1016/j.nic.2022.02.004
1052-5149/22/© 2022 Elsevier Inc. All rights reserved.

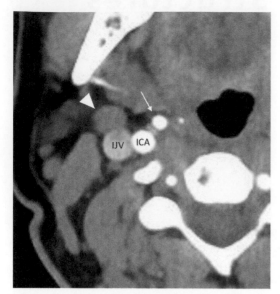

Fig. 1. Axial computed tomography angiogram (CTA) neck image shows some contents of the carotid sheath, the ICA, ECA (*arrow*), and IJV. There is also a lymph node (*arrowhead*).

The CCAs continue cephalad until they bifurcate, each into an ICA and an ECA (Fig. 3). The bifurcation is usually located at the level of the superior border of the thyroid cartilage at around C3-C4[1] or at the level of the hyoid bone.[5]

Internal carotid arteries

The proximal ICA is dilated and called the carotid bulb (see Fig. 3).[1] Like the CCA, the cervical, or extracranial, ICA usually does not have branches.[6]

As the ICA proceeds intracranially into the skull base through the carotid canal into the petrous segment (Fig. 4A), branches appear, such as the caroticotympanic and vidian arteries. The cavernous segment of the ICA (Fig. 4B) begins as the vessel passes through the dura at the cavernous sinus. Although not generally visible on cross-sectional imaging, there are trunks along the cavernous segment, some of which provide supply to the pituitary gland. When the ICA passes

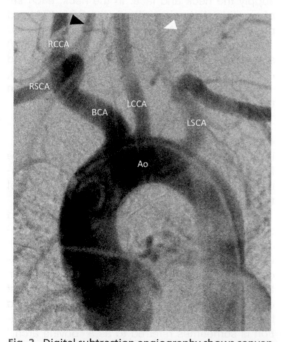

Fig. 2. Digital subtraction angiography shows conventional aortic arch (Ao) anatomy. The first branch is the brachiocephalic artery (BCA), from which the right CCA (RCCA) and right subclavian artery (RSCA) branch. The second branch of the arch is the left CCA (LCCA). The third is the left SCA (LSCA). The right vertebral artery (VA) (*black arrowhead*) and left VA (*white arrowhead*) are faintly seen, each originating from their respective SCA.

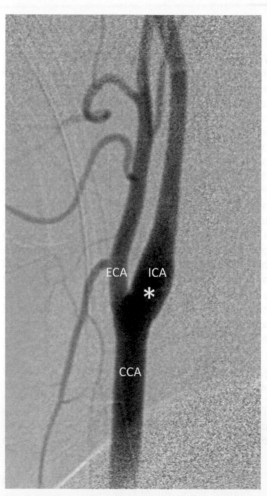

Fig. 3. Digital subtraction angiography shows the CCA bifurcating into the ICA and ECA. The carotid bulb is marked with an *asterisk*.

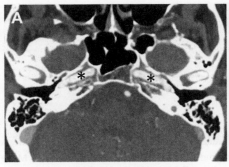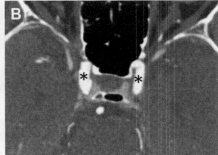

Fig. 4. Axial CTA shows (A) petrous and (B) cavernous segments of the intracranial ICAs (asterisks).

through the roof of the cavernous sinus, it becomes the supraclinoid segment, which has branches and terminates as the anterior and medial cerebral arteries (not further discussed).[6]

External carotid arteries

Although the main role of the ICA is to supply the intracranial circulation, the ECA (see Fig. 3) and its many branches (Box 1) supply the face and scalp. The branches are named after the territories they supply.[7] There are many anastomoses among ECA branches including with contralateral ones. They also provide anastomoses to the intracranial circulation (eg, if there is occlusion of the intracranial ICA). Blood flow between anastomoses may go in either direction.[6]

Vertebral arteries

Although the carotid arteries supply the intracranial anterior circulation, the vertebral arteries (VA) supply the intracranial posterior circulation.[8]

The right VA originates from the right subclavian artery (see Fig. 2), which is the second branch of the brachiocephalic artery distal to the right CCA. The left VA classically originates from the left subclavian artery (see Fig. 2), the third branch of the aortic arch. These arteries are located deep to the longus colli and anterior scalene muscles of

---

Box 1
External carotid artery branches

- Superior thyroid artery
- Ascending pharyngeal artery
- Lingual artery
- Facial artery
- Occipital artery
- Posterior auricular artery
- Superficial temporal artery
- Internal maxillary artery

---

the neck (Fig. 5A) until they enter the transverse foramina of the cervical vertebrae (Fig. 5B), usually at the C6 level. The VAs then travel superiorly though the transverse foramina of the cervical spine. At C1 the vessels bend posteriorly and medially (Fig. 5C). At the craniocervical junction, the vessels enter the foramen magnum, through the dura, and become intracranial (see Fig. 5C).[6] Some choose to describe parts of the VA by dividing it into four segments (V1-V4) (Box 2).[9] There may be anastomoses with ECA branches and other arteries and there are small branches of the cervical segment that supply the vertebral bodies and neck musculature.[6] Meningeal branches near the foramen magnum supply the skull and falx cerebelli.[8] The VAs can decrease in caliber when they become intracranial.[10] The VAs, in their intracranial portions, also provide some arterial supply to the spinal cord, in addition to the brain.

Veins of Head and Neck

The jugular venous system, veins of the face, and the vertebral venous system are the main venous pathways that are described. The IJVs are major conduits that bring venous blood from the head to the heart. An additional means to return venous blood from the head is through the vertebral venous system. Other venous structures that are mentioned are the inferior petrosal sinus (IPS) and the emissary veins at the skull base, which are interrelated with the IJV and/or vertebral venous system.

Internal jugular vein

The right and left IJVs drain intracerebral blood, each receiving a sigmoid sinus which is the main terminal dural venous sinus of the head. The IJVs receive blood from other veins of the skull, face, and neck as they course inferiorly through the neck.[1]

The proximal or superior portion of each IJV is located at the skull base and is called the jugular bulb, where the vessel dilates and receives blood

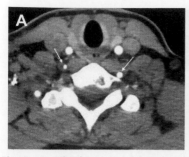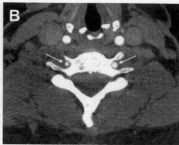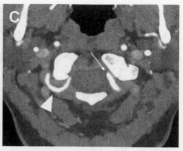

Fig. 5. Vertebral arteries. (*A*) Axial CTA neck shows V1 segments (*arrows*) in the lower neck. (*B*) More superiorly, V2 segments (*arrows*) are situated within transverse foramina. (*C*) Right VA (RVA) V3 segment (*arrowhead*) at the C1 level bending into the spinal canal, still extradural. The V4 segment is just beginning for the left VA (LVA) (*arrow*), as it crosses the dura.

from the sigmoid sinus (**Fig. 6**A). The jugular bulbs are located within the jugular foramina at the skull base (**Fig. 6**B), more specifically in the pars vascularis with the vagus (CN X) and spinal accessory (CN XI) nerves. Of note, the jugular bulb is normally located along to the hypotympanum of the middle ear and a bony jugular plate separates the middle ear from the bulb (see **Fig 6**B).[11]

As the IJV descends through the neck, it is located in the carotid sheath (see **Fig. 1**). In the upper chest, each IJV joins with a subclavian vein (SCV) to form a brachiocephalic vein (BCV) (**Fig. 7**). The right and left BCVs drain into the superior vena cava, which then drains into the right atrium of the heart. Other veins from the head and neck variably drain into the IJV. Also at the inferior end of the IJV, there is an inferior bulb, which is a dilated segment located above valves.[1] Valves also are present in the SCVs in variable locations, most toward the half approaching the BCVs.[12]

Veins of face and neck

There are numerous veins of the neck and face that eventually drain into the external jugular vein (EJV) and IJV. Because there are so many veins and variant interconnections, the more commonly mentioned veins and their conventional configurations are covered. Discussion centers around the

anterior facial vein (AFV), posterior facial vein (PFV) with its anterior (ABPFV) and posterior branches (PBPFV), EJV, and anterior jugular vein (AJV).

Supraorbital and supratrochlear veins located above the orbits and at the forehead drain into the angular vein.[13] At the root, or top, of the nose, the angular vein becomes the anterior facial vein (AFV).[6,14] The AFV continues inferiorly along the side of the nose, anterior to the maxillary sinus, and then to the lateral aspect of the submandibular gland (**Fig. 8**). In some sources the angular vein and AFV together are called the facial vein, with the superior most portion being called the angular vein.[13] On a practical note, the AFV, when identifiable, may be used as a landmark to determine if a facial mass is within or external to the submandibular gland.[14] The AFV is revisited later.

There are several superficial veins draining the head and scalp that form a network. Some tributaries of this network form the superficial temporal vein[9] on the side of the face above the zygomatic arch. Additional veins drain into the superficial temporal vein, such as the parotid veins and the middle temporal vein, which drains the orbital vein.[9] Within the parotid gland, the superficial temporal vein joins the internal maxillary vein to form the PFV, also commonly called the retromandibular vein (**Fig. 9**A).[14,15] Of note, the PFV is located between the ECA and facial nerve.[9] The PFV divides into the anterior branch of the posterior facial vein (ABPFV) and the posterior branch of the facial vein (PBPFV) in the parotid gland (**Fig. 9**B).[14]

The ABPFV extends inferiorly to the posterior aspect of the submandibular gland to connect to the AFV (**Fig. 10**A), to form the common facial vein (**Fig. 10**B). The common facial vein drains into the IJV sometimes around the mandibular angle (**Fig. 10**C).[15]

The PBPFV joins the posterior auricular vein (see **Fig. 9**A, B; **Fig. 11**A), which arises from a

---

Box 2
Vertebral artery segments

- V1: Origin to C6 before transverse foramen
- V2: C6 transverse foramen to C2 transverse foramen
- V3: C2 above transverse foramen to extradural spinal canal above C1
- V4: Entrance to dura at craniocervical junction, intracranial

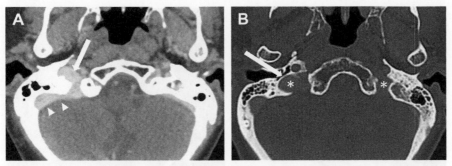

Fig. 6. (*A*) Axial contrast-enhanced CT (CECT) at the skull base level shows the right sigmoid sinus (*arrowheads*) draining into the right jugular bulb (*arrow*). (*B*) *Asterisks* are located within bilateral jugular bulbs in this axial bone algorithm CT image. The right is larger than the left. The right jugular plate is denoted by the *arrow*.

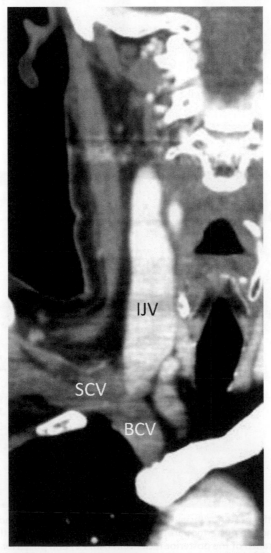

Fig. 7. CECT neck shows the opacified right IJV draining into the unopacified right SCV, to form the right BCV.

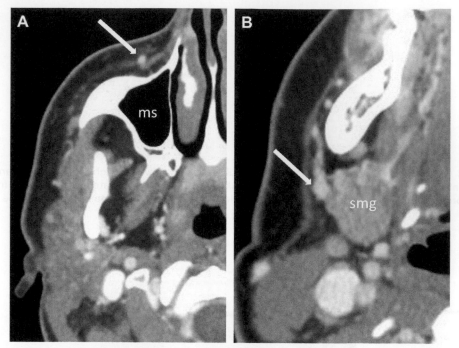

Fig. 8. (*A*) Axial CECT image shows the anterior facial vein (AFV) (*arrow*) at the level of the maxillary sinus (ms). (*B*) The AFV (*arrow*) continues inferiorly along the submandibular gland (smg).

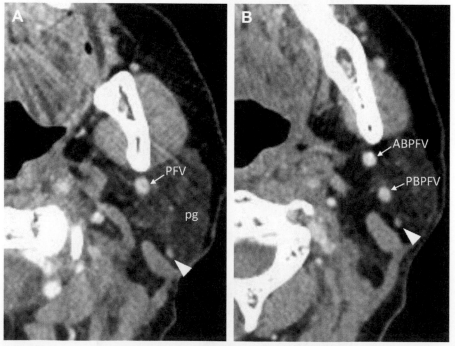

Fig. 9. (*A*) Axial CECT shows the posterior facial vein (PFV) within the parotid gland (pg). The posterior auricular vein (*arrowhead*) is seen along the posterior parotid gland. (*B*) More inferiorly in the parotid gland, the PFV has branched into the anterior branch of the posterior facial vein (ABPFV) and posterior branch of the posterior facial vein (PBPFV). The posterior auricular vein (*arrowhead*) approaches closer to the PBPFV.

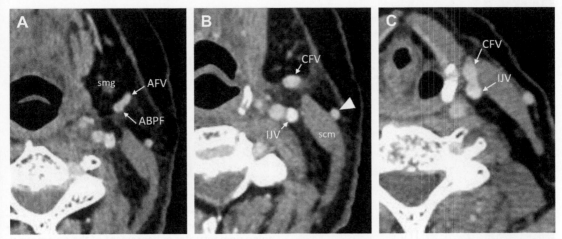

Fig. 10. (*A*) CECT CT neck shows anterior facial vein (AFV) and anterior branch of the posterior facial vein (ABPFV) joining next to a fat-replaced submandibular gland (smg). (*B*) More inferiorly the common facial vein (CFV) has formed from the AFV and ABPFV. The external jugular vein (EJV) is present lateral to the sternocleidomastoid muscle (scm). The internal jugular vein (IJV) is noted. (*C*) More inferiorly, the CFV drains into the IJV.

parietooccipital venous network in the scalp, becoming the EJV in or below the parotid gland (**Fig. 11**B, C).[13,14]

The EJV extends inferiorly in the neck, superficial and lateral to the sternocleidomastoid muscle (see **Fig. 10**B). It terminates most commonly at the confluence of the IJV and SCV (**Fig. 12**), and less commonly at the SCV or the IJV.[14,15] Other veins, such as the AJV, may drain into the EJV and there may be a branch between the IJV and EJV at the parotid gland.[1]

In the anterior neck above the level of the hyoid bone, superficial veins and connections from the facial veins and IJV drain into the AJV (**Fig. 13**).

There are usually two, although there may be only one, which course near the midline of the neck, anterior to the sternocleidomastoid muscles.[1,14,15] These terminate at the SCV or EJV. There may be a jugular venous arch (or transverse jugular arch) bridging the right and left AJVs. Other veins may communicate with the AJV and the jugular venous arch.[14,15]

Venous Structures of the Skull Base

Various smaller venous sinuses and emissary veins at the skull base receive drainage from the major dural venous sinuses and face, with interconnections to the cavernous sinuses and IPS.

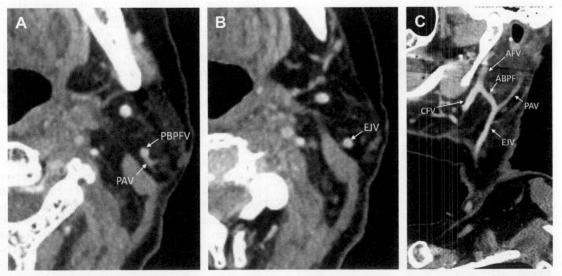

Fig. 11. (*A*) CECT neck shows the posterior branch of the posterior facial vein (PBPFV) joining the posterior auricular vein (PAV). (*B*) Inferiorly, external jugular vein (EJV) has formed. (*C*) Sagittal reformatted perspective of the formation of the EJV, with additional anatomy noted.

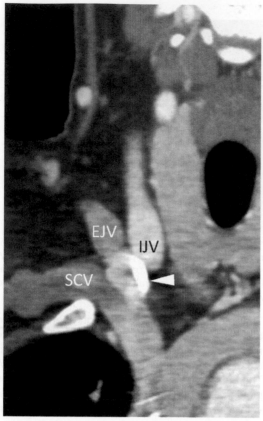

Fig. 12. Coronal reformatted CECT neck shows EJV draining into the confluence of the IJV and SCV. Part of a central venous access catheter is seen at the confluence (*arrowhead*).

These venous structures provide connections to the vertebral venous system or to other extracranial venous structures.

Cavernous sinuses
The cavernous sinuses (**Fig. 14**) are venous plexuses seen on both sides of the sella and

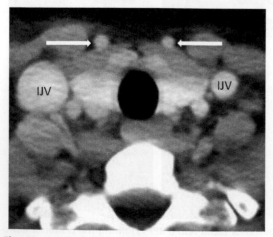

Fig. 13. Axial CECT neck shows the anterior jugular veins (*arrows*). Internal jugular veins (IJV) are noted.

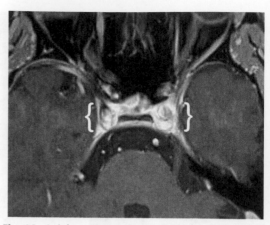

Fig. 14. Axial contrast-enhanced (CE) T1 VIBE MR imaging demonstrates enhancement of the cavernous sinuses (*brackets*).

connected to each other by intercavernous sinuses and the basilar plexus. They are valveless with reversible flow, and the ICAs and cranial nerves IV, V1, V2, and VI pass through them. Multiple venous structures communicate with the cavernous sinus, including superior and inferior ophthalmic veins, IPS and superior petrosal sinus, and superficial middle cerebral veins.[16]

Inferior petrosal sinuses
The cavernous sinuses drain into the IPS (**Fig. 15A, B**). The IPS receives other veins and is connected to the basilar plexus and superior petrosal sinus. The IPS is located along the posterior and inferior aspects of the cavernous sinuses, along the petroclival fissures, and continues into the jugular foramina where they connect with the jugular bulbs (see **Fig. 15B**). They sometimes drain through the hypoglossal canals into the suboccipital venous plexus.[16]

Emissary veins
Various emissary veins provide a connection between intracranial venous sinuses and extracranial venous structures, importantly the vertebral venous system, at the skull base. These veins traverse cranial foramina and canals and may be variably present. Anatomy and interconnections among these intracranial, emissary, and extracranial venous structures is complex. This anatomy has been described in the literature by San Millan Ruiz and colleagues[17] as "fragmentary and incomplete" because of technically difficult anatomic dissection of these structures and that supine positioning on venography may not give a complete picture. Some emissary veins are the mastoid (**Fig. 16**), posterior condylar (condylar emissary) (**Fig. 17**), anterior condylar (venous plexus of the hypoglossal nerve) (see **Fig. 17**),

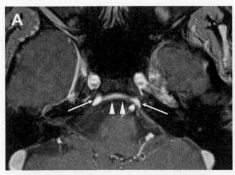
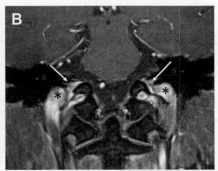

Fig. 15. (*A*) Axial CE T1 VIBE MR imaging inferior to the level of the cavernous sinuses shows enhancement of the IPS (*arrows*) and basilar plexus (*arrowheads*). (*B*) Coronal image demonstrates the left and right IPS (*arrows*) draining into ipsilateral jugular bulbs (*asterisks*).

and lateral condylar veins. Simplified, the anterior condylar veins lead to the internal vertebral venous plexus (IVVP), whereas the posterior and lateral condylar veins feed into components of the external vertebral venous system.[17]

Vertebral Venous System

Besides the IJVs, a lesser known means to drain venous blood from the head to the heart is through the vertebral venous system. This drainage occurs through a series of interconnected veins and venous plexuses. The start of these connections begins intracranially via the venous sinuses and jugular bulbs, through emissary veins, which then connect to the vertebral venous system. It has

been described that when upright, the main venous drainage path from the brain is through the vertebral venous plexus, whereas the IJV is the main drainage path from the brain when supine.[17]

There is a wide array of descriptions and nomenclature used for the vertebral venous system. The following description is simplified from various descriptions and covers the portion at the neck. There is an IVVP (**Fig. 18**), referring to structures within the spinal canal. There is an anterior IVVP situated between two layers of the posterior longitudinal ligament[18] and an epidural posterior IVVP. The other component of the vertebral venous system is the external vertebral venous plexus, referring to structures outside of the spinal canal (see **Figs. 18**; **Fig. 19**). These include the vertebral artery venous plexus (see

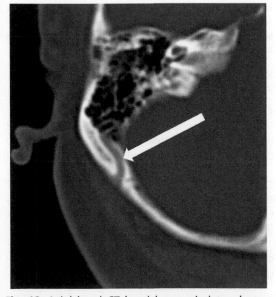

Fig. 16. Axial head CT head bone windows show a vascular channel through the skull for the mastoid emissary vein (*arrow*), which drains from the sigmoid sinus into the suboccipital venous plexus (not shown).

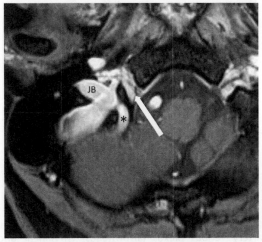

Fig. 17. CE T1 VIBE MR imaging shows a posterior emissary vein (*asterisk*) draining posteriorly from the jugular bulb (JB). Anterior emissary veins travel through the hypoglossal canal (*arrow*).

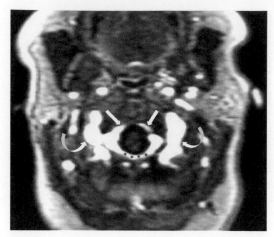

Fig. 18. Axial reformatted CE MR venogram at the level of C1 shows opacification within the extradural spinal canal, specifically the anterior internal vertebral venous plexus (*arrows*) and posterior internal vertebral venous plexus (*asterisks*). Various components of the external vertebral venous plexus (EVVP) opacify In the paraspinal soft tissues.

Fig. 19)[17] and the vertebral vein (**Fig. 20**), which sometimes is seen coursing inferiorly from C6 into the BCV at the junction of the SCV and IJV.[14] Connections exist between the external and internal venous systems, such as through the intervertebral veins.[17]

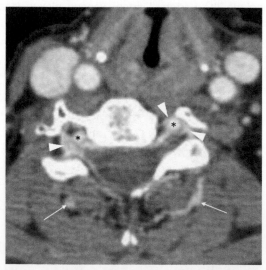

Fig. 19. Axial CECT neck demonstrates the vertebral artery venous plexus (*arrowheads*) curvilinear and amorphous enhancement, located around the VAs (*asterisks*). Other components of the external vertebral venous plexus are present in the paraspinal soft tissues (*arrows*).

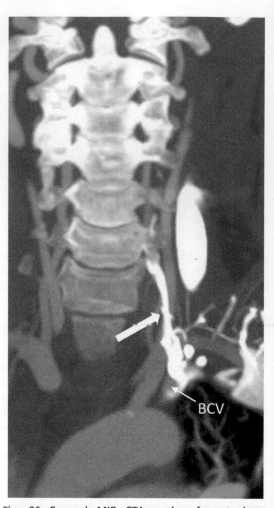

Fig. 20. Coronal MIP CTA neck reformat shows contrast refluxed into the left vertebral vein (*arrow*), seen exiting the left C6 neural foramen and draining inferiorly into the BCV.

VARIANTS AND DISEASE MIMICS
Arteries

Cervical carotid arteries
Variable branches, location, absence, and morphology are some of the more commonly described anatomic variants of the CCAs.

Anomalous branches: Rare branching from the CCA and cervical ICA, such as vertebral, superior thyroid, and superior laryngeal arteries[6,9] from the CCA, and VA[19] and ECA branches[20] from the ICA (**Fig. 21**).

Carotid bifurcation level: May be inferior or superior to the typical C3-C4 or hyoid level. Surgeons may use position as landmark.

Absent ICA: Developmental agenesis or aplasia.

○ Agenesis: complete lack of development.[21]
○ Aplasia: lack of normal visible vessel, with evidence of some previous development, such

as remnants seen in surgery or bony carotid canal on imaging (**Fig. 22**).[21]

○ Various anastomoses compensate for an absent ICA. May be important to delineate for surgical or endovascular treatment planning. For example, an intracavernous anastomotic vessel could be injured during transphenoidal surgery.[21]

○ Clues to differentiate developmental absence from occlusion include lack of carotid canal, small canal, and anastomoses.

○ Possible increased risk of aneurysm with absent ICA. Surveillance imaging could be considered.[21]

Hypoplasia: Incomplete development resulting in diffusely small caliber vessel.[21] Hypoplasia is differentiated from stenosis or dissection by presence of small carotid canal.

Cervical ICA fenestration and duplication: This is rare. Duplications also may be an ICA paired with an aberrant ICA. Gailloud and colleagues[22] angiographic case series raised the possibility that cervical ICA fenestrations may be dissections. Careful evaluation of vessel morphology is suggested.

Persistent embryonic carotid-vertebrobasilar anastomoses: Vessels connecting the vertebrobasilar system and ICA. Two types involving the cervical ICA are rare.

○ Persistent proatlantal artery type 1: Vertebrobasilar system to ICA at the level of C2 or C3.[23]

○ Persistent hypoglossal artery: Vertebrobasilar system to ICA at the level of C1 or C1-C2 interspace (**Fig. 23**).[23]

Retropharyngeal ICAs: May be unilateral or bilateral. In some individuals, carotid arteries change to and from retropharyngeal position

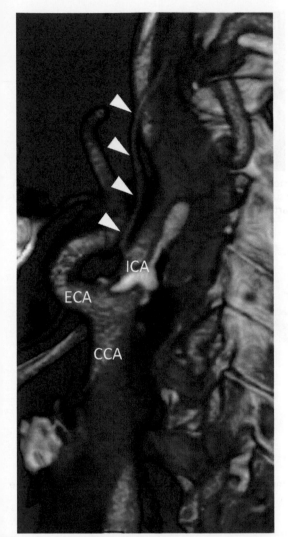

Fig. 21. Three-dimensional reformatted CTA neck near the carotid bifurcation demonstrates an anomalous occipital artery (*arrowheads*) originating from the ICA.

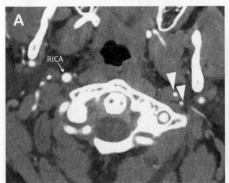
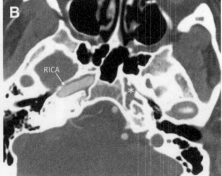

Fig. 22. (*A*) Axial CTA image demonstrates an absent left ICA and normal right ICA (RICA). Enhancing vessels on the left (*arrowheads*) are left external carotid artery branches. (*B*) A rudimentary carotid canal (*asterisk*) may be present, suggesting aplasia of the left ICA.

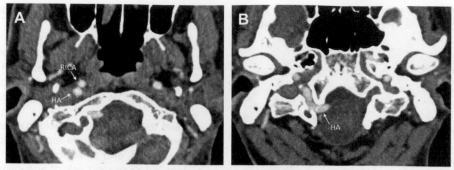

Fig. 23. (*A*) Below the skull base, axial CTA shows a persistent hypoglossal artery (HA) posterolateral to the RICA, from which it had branched at the level of C2. (*B*) More superiorly the artery (HA) travels through the right hypoglossal canal, becomes intradural. It joins the basilar artery (not shown).

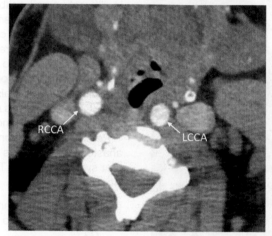

Fig. 24. Axial CTA neck shows a retropharyngeal LCCA impressing on the posterior pharynx, in contrast to the typical position of the RCCA.

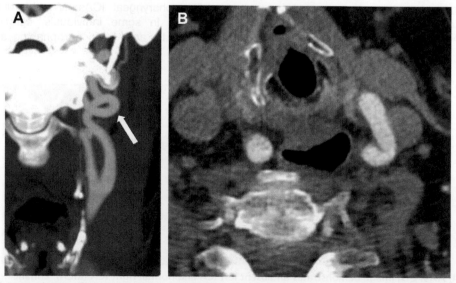

Fig. 25. (*A*) Coronal MIP reformatted CTA image shows a tortuous cervical left ICA (*arrow*). (*B*) Axial CTA image of a different patient demonstrates kinking of the left CCA.

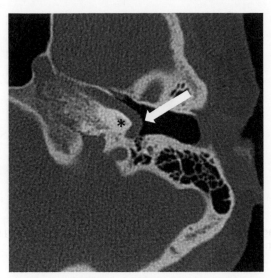

Fig. 26. Axial temporal bone CT shows the inferior tympanic-caroticotympanic anastomosis (*arrow*) over the cochlear promontory (*asterisk*) in a patient with an aberrant ICA.

(Fig. 24).[24] Retropharyngeal carotid arteries can present as a retropharyngeal mass that should not be biopsied, and potentially complicate head and neck surgery[24] or anterior approach spine surgery.[25]

Morphologic variants: Includes tortuosity, kinking, or coiling (Fig. 25). Can be seen in other arteries. May make diagnosis of stenosis or other vascular abnormality more difficult.[26]

Intracranial internal carotid artery
Aberrant ICA and lateralized petrous ICA: Two rare variants in which ICA protrudes into middle ear cavity. ICA is susceptible to injury during temporal bone surgery.

○ Aberrant ICA: Normally, a small caroticotympanic artery passes into the middle ear and anastomoses with a small inferior tympanic artery. With aberrant ICA, there is an "under-developed" ICA[27] and caroticotympanic and inferior tympanic arteries form an enlarged anastomosis that passes over the cochlear prominence, projecting into the middle ear (Fig. 26). Associated with a persistent stapedial artery that becomes the middle meningeal artery and absent foramen spinosum.[27,28]

○ Lateralized petrous ICA: Genu of the petrous ICA extends more laterally than expected, protrudes into anterior mesotympanum. Can have thin or dehiscent lateral wall. Computed

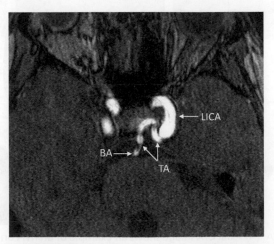

Fig. 27. Three-dimensional time-of-flight MR angiography of the head shows a tortuous persistent trigeminal artery (TA) connecting the cavernous left ICA (LICA) with the basilar artery (BA).

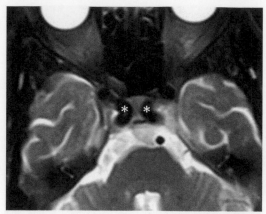

Fig. 28. T2-weighted MR imaging of the brain demonstrates flow voids of "kissing carotid arteries" (*asterisks*) at the level of the cavernous sinuses.

tomography (CT), for its ability to delineate bony landmarks, is considered best for diagnosis and differentiation from an aberrant ICA.[28]

Persistent embryonic carotid-vertebrobasilar anastomoses involving intracranial ICA:

○ Trigeminal artery: Vertebrobasilar system to cavernous ICA. Most common of these anastomoses (Fig. 27).[29]
○ Otic artery: Vertebrobasilar system to petrous ICA via internal auditory canal; rare.[29]

Kissing carotid arteries (Fig. 28): Both cavernous ICAs with medial course appear to

contact or nearly contact. This may complicate transphenoidal pituitary surgery.[30]

External carotid arteries
Variant branch anatomy: Many variations and anastomoses.[6]
   Absent ECA: Rare.[7]

Vertebral arteries
When the VA is not seen where it is expected, it may be mistaken for an occluded vessel. If there is size asymmetry, one must differentiate between a pathologic stenosis or normal vessel.
   Variant origins: Examples include the left VA originating directly from the aortic arch between

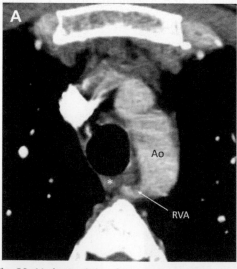
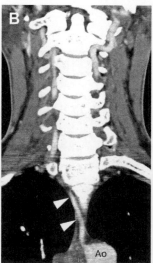
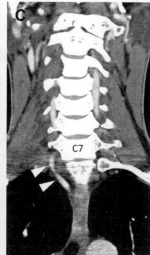

Fig. 29. Variant origin of RVA. (*A*) Axial CTA image shows an example of an RVA originating from the aortic arch (Ao), distal to the left SCA. The RVA is traversing posterior to the esophagus (*asterisk*). (*B, C*) The vessel (*arrowheads*) is shown on its way to the right neck and enters the right C7 transverse foramen.

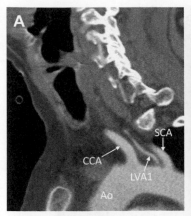
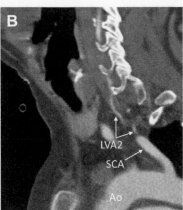
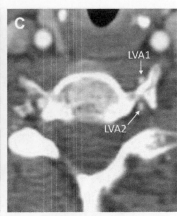

Fig. 30. Duplicate origins of vertebral artery. (A) CTA oblique sagittal reformat shows one moiety of the left VA (LVA1) originating directly from the aortic arch between the left CCA and left SCA. (B) The second left VA moiety originates from the left SCA. Both moieties are small in caliber. (C) Axial view at the level of C6 shows one moiety of the left VA has entered the C6 transverse foramen. Both moieties join shortly above (not shown).

the brachiocephalic and left subclavian origins (most common) or arising distal to the left subclavian artery.[31] Variant origins of right VA are less frequent (Fig. 29).[32]

Duplicate origins: Also may see combinations of duplicate and anomalous origins (Fig. 30).[32] Duplicated vessels tend to be small in caliber, which may complicate catheter angiography or be mistaken for dissections.[33]

Level of entry into the transverse foramina: Normally at C6. Reported at levels from C2-C7 (Fig. 31).[34]

Asymmetry: More commonly, one VA is dominant or larger than the other (Fig. 32), although is similar in caliber or codominant.[6] Small nondominant vessels may be mistaken for dissection or stenosis. Conversely dissection may be mistaken

for a normal, small VA.[35] Luminal contour irregularities or T1 shortening from intramural hematoma on MR imaging or MR angiogram suggest dissection. Correlation with size of transverse foramina or comparison with prior vascular imaging also may be helpful.

Hypoplasia: Various criteria, such as diameter less than 2 to 2.5 mm (see Fig. 32).[36]

Fenestration: Considered rare by some. May be mistaken for dissection (Fig. 33).[37]

Veins

Internal jugular veins

Jugular foramina asymmetry: Asymmetry (see Fig. 6) sometimes may cause concern for pathology, including skull metastasis or paraganglioma.

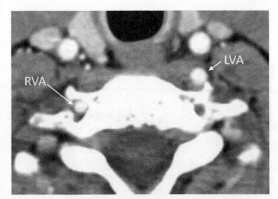

Fig. 31. Asymmetric level of entry into transverse foramina. RVA within the right C7 transverse foramen, the left transverse foramen is empty. The LVA is anterior to the transverse process and enters the transverse foramina at C6.

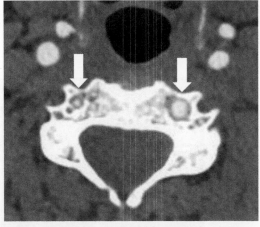

Fig. 32. Axial CTA neck shows asymmetry of the VAs (arrows). The right VA is hypoplastic. Note the sizes of the transverse foramina, which are commensurate to the size of the VAs.

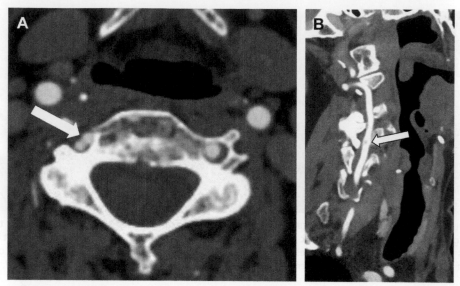

Fig. 33. (A) Axial CTA neck image shows right VA fenestration (arrow). In isolation, this single image could be confused for dissection, pseudoaneurysm, or duplication of the VA (B) Oblique sagittal reformat demonstrates short segment fenestration (arrow).

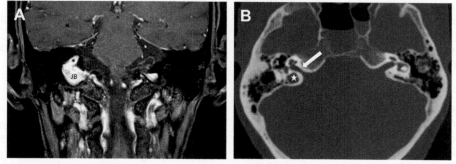

Fig. 34. (A) Coronal CE T1 VIBE MR image shows a superiorly directed outpouching, compatible with a diverticulum (asterisk), from the right jugular bulb (JB). (B) Axial CT demonstrates that this same jugular bulb with diverticulum (star) is high-riding, seen at the level of the internal auditory canal (arrow).

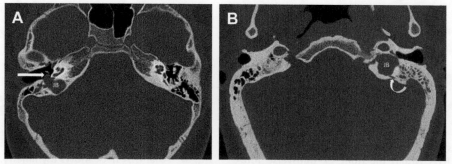

Fig. 35. (A) Bone algorithm axial CT shows a right JB with a diverticulum demonstrating an area of dehiscence (arrow) that projects into the right middle ear. (B) Bone algorithm axial CT shows left jugular bulb dehiscent with a left vestibular aqueduct (curved arrow).

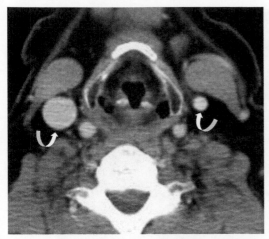

Fig. 36. Axial CECT shows asymmetric internal jugular veins (*curved arrows*).

On CT, smooth and round borders rather than irregular edges characterize a normal jugular foramen.[11]

High jugular bulb: Various definitions, including when the superior border of bulb is at or above the level of internal auditory canal (**Fig. 34**). This can be a surgical risk. Overlying bone may be dehiscent or thin.[38]

Dehiscent jugular bulb: Absent bony plate between bulb and middle ear (**Fig. 35**). Can be

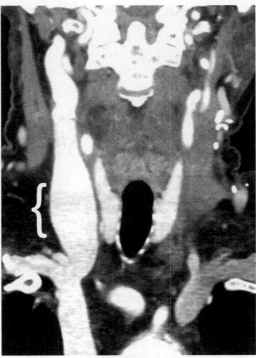

Fig. 38. Axial reformatted CECT neck shows phlebectasia (*bracket*) at the inferior end of the right IJV.

associated with high jugular bulb. Also may have dehiscence next to vestibular aqueduct (**Fig. 35**).[39]

Jugular diverticulum: Variant outpouching from jugular bulb (see **Fig. 34**A, B). Well-corticated margins on CT.[40] Flow contiguous with jugular bulb on vascular imaging. Diverticuli may point in different directions into petrous bone, less commonly into occipital condyle.[40,41]

IJV asymmetry: Right is IJV often larger than the left (**Fig. 36**),[42–44] although can be codominant.

Indentations of the IJV: Because of vein compressibility, sometimes IJV is indented by transverse process of C1,[15,44] styloid process (**Fig. 37**),[44] or lower in the neck by the ICA[15,44] and posterior belly of the digastric muscle.[44] Jayaraman and colleagues[44] described only 35% of patients in their CTA series had upper jugular veins without significant extrinsic compression and that it was unclear or unlikely that there is physiologic significance, although others have made associations of venous compression with other conditions.

Valves: Most patients have an IJV valve. Can be located inferior to the jugular bulb[15] or near inferior end of IJV.[14] Valves may give false appearance of stenosis.[45]

Phlebectasia: Focal dilatation of IJV inferior to the valve at the inferior end of vessel (**Fig. 38**). Phlebectasia may be mistaken for aneurysm.[14]

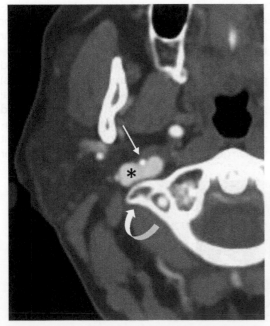

Fig. 37. Styloid process (*thin arrow*) and the transverse process of C1 (*curved arrow*) indent the upper right internal jugular vein (*asterisk*).

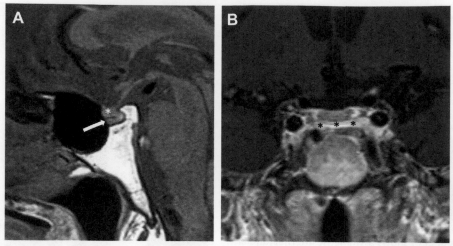

Fig. 39. Intercavernous sinus. (A) Sagittal T1-weighted image of the sella shows an unenhanced intercavernous sinus (arrow) inferior to the pituitary gland (asterisk), which could be concerning for a lesion. (B) CE coronal T1-weighted image of the sella shows enhancement across the inferior aspect of the sella, consistent with an intercavernous sinus (asterisks).

Other: Variable IJV size including hypoplasia (<5.45 mm per Lim and colleagues[42] CT series), duplication,[15] and fenestration.[46]

Veins of face and neck

Variant anatomy: Variable drainage of superficial veins of the face and EJVs.[15]

Duplicated EJVs: Considered rare.[47]

Cavernous sinuses

Varying amounts of fat and fibrous tissue: Also varying flow. May result in variable appearances and asymmetry on MR imaging and CT scan.[48]

Dilated intercavernous sinus (Fig. 39): Mimics mass along sellar floor on MR imaging. Considered a normal variant, also is more prominent with intracranial hypotension.[49]

Emissary veins

Asymmetry: Bony canal asymmetry at skull base or absence of venous channels. In the hypoglossal canal, may see emissary vein enhancement or

nonenhancing cerebrospinal fluid signal or density.[50]

Miscellaneous

Pterygoid venous plexus: Located around the pterygoid muscles at the skull base (Fig. 40). Various emissary veins connect cavernous sinuses to pterygoid venous plexus.[16] Pterygoid venous plexus drains into internal maxillary veins.[6,14] Streaky hyperintense signal on T2-weighted imaging or enhancement on contrast-enhanced MR imaging or CT may be irregular[6] or asymmetric and mistaken for a vascular malformation.

Pharyngolaryngeal venous plexuses: Found posterior to the laryngeal (postcricoid plexus) (Fig. 41) or hypopharyngeal (posterior pharyngeal plexus) mucosa. Described in patients with head and neck cancer and lymphoma. On CT, submucosal enhancement matching density of adjacent veins, generally a few millimeters thick. May or

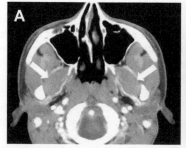
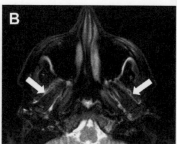
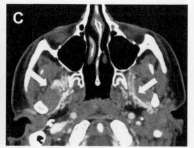

Fig. 40. Pterygoid venous plexus variable enhancement and signal in different patients. (A) CECT shows streaky symmetric enhancement (arrows). (B) T2-weighted MR imaging demonstrates streaky hyperintense signal (arrows). (C) CECT shows asymmetric enhancement (arrows).

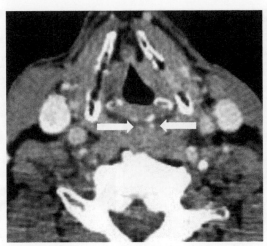

Fig. 41. CE CT neck of a patient with head and neck cancer, status post chemoradiation therapy. Small foci of enhancement (*between arrows*) posterior to the cricoid are compatible with a postcricoid venous plexus, a subset of pharyngolaryngeal venous plexus.

may not be present on baseline imaging, but can appear on follow-up and be confused for tumor.[51]

Carotid body: Chemoreceptor that helps regulate blood pressure and respiration. Located at carotid bifurcation in adventitia. Sometimes seen on CT as subcentimeter ovoid enhancing focus, at inferomedial carotid bifurcation (**Fig. 42**). Differentiation between normal carotid body and small paraganglioma (glomus tumor) may be difficult. Lesion measuring greater than

6 mm (± 2 standard deviation) may require further investigation.[52]

Thoracic duct: Part of the lymphatic system, carries lymph toward heart. Left thoracic duct and right lymphatic duct (also called right thoracic duct) drain into the angle formed at ipsilateral IJV and SCV confluence.[53] Left is more commonly visible on imaging, appears as round or tubular structures (**Fig. 43**), and may be mistaken for enlarged or cystic lymph nodes and other lesions.[54]

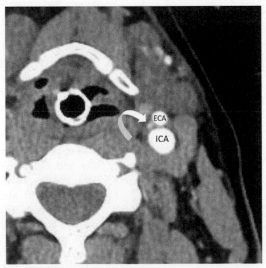

Fig. 42. CTA neck demonstrates a tiny enhancing focus, likely a carotid body (*arrow*), located between the left ICA and ECA.

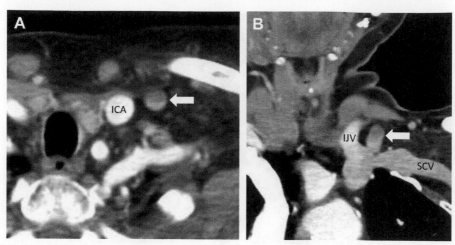

Fig. 43. (*A*) Axial CECT neck shows thoracic duct (*arrow*). (*B*) Coronal reformat demonstrates thoracic duct (*arrow*) draining into confluence of left IJV and left SCV.

SUMMARY

Normal anatomy of the arteries and veins of the head and neck and their appearance on imaging may sometimes be simple and sometimes complex. Familiarity with normal anatomy and variants can help one differentiate normal findings from disease mimics. Variants are problematic for surgical or angiographic procedures, and recognition of them can help with planning and potentially avoiding complications.

CLINICS CARE POINTS

- Arterial and venous systems in the neck serve to supply and provide drainage for the brain, in addition to the face and neck.

- Vascular variants in the neck may mimic pathology and awareness of their appearances may help one make diagnoses or avoid potential pitfalls for angiographic or surgical procedures.

DISCLOSURE

The authors report no relevant disclosures.

REFERENCES

1. Watkinson JC, Gleeson M. Neck. In: Standring S, editor. In: gray's anatomy: the anatomic basis of clinical practice. 42nd edition. Philadelphia: Elsevier; 2020. p. 573–606.e1.

2. Chengazi HU, Bhatt AA. Pathology of the carotid space. Insights Imaging 2019;10(1):21.

3. Ahn SS, Chen SW, Miller TJ, et al. What is the true incidence of anomalous bovine left common carotid artery configuration? Ann Vasc Surg 2014;28(2):381–5.

4. Layton KF, Kallmes DF, Cloft HJ, et al. Bovine aortic arch variant in humans: clarification of a common misnomer. Am J Neuroradiol 2006;27:1541–2.

5. Lo A, Oehley M, Bartlett A, et al. Anatomical variations of the common carotid artery bifurcation. ANZ J Surg 2006;76(11):970–2.

6. Johnson MH, Thorisson HM, Diluna ML. Vascular anatomy: the head, neck, and skull base. Neurosurg Clin N Am 2009;20(3):239–58.

7. Thurlow PC, Andrus JM, Wholey MH. Common cervical and cerebral vascular variants. Interv Cardiol Clin 2014;3(1):123–34.

8. Conesa Bertran G, Delgado-Martinez I. Vascular supply and drainage of the brain. In: Standring S, editor. Gray's anatomy: the anatomic basis of clinical practice. 42nd edition. Philadelphia: Elsevier; 2020. p. 415–24.e1.

9. Standring S. The anatomy of the vascular and lymphatic systems. In: Standring S, editor. Gray's anatomy: the anatomic basis of clinical practice. 42nd edition. Philadelphia: Elsevier; 2020. p. 1464.e6-12.

10. Woraputtaporn W, Ananteerakul T, Iamsaard S, et al. Incidence of vertebral artery of aortic arch origin, its level of entry into transverse foramen, length, diameter and clinical significance. Anat Sci Int 2019;94(4):275–9.

11. Caldemeyer KS, Mathews VP, Azzarelli B, et al. The jugular foramen: a review of anatomy, masses, and imaging characteristics. Radiographics 1997;17(5):1123–39.

12. Celepci H, Brenner E. Position of valves within the subclavian and axillary veins. J Vasc Surg 2011;54(6 Suppl):70S-6S.

13. Holmes S. Face and scalp. In: Standring S, editor. Gray's anatomy: the anatomic basis of clinical practice. 42nd edition. Philadelphia: Elsevier; 2020. p. 607–35.e1.

14. Escott EJ, Branstetter BF. It's not a cervical lymph node, it's a vein: CT and MR imaging findings in the veins of the head and neck. Radiographics 2006;26(5):1501–15.

15. Werner JD, Siskin GP, Mandato K, et al. Review of venous anatomy for venographic interpretation in chronic cerebrospinal venous insufficiency. J Vasc Interv Radiol 2011;22(12):1681–90. quiz 1691.

16. Bhangoo RS, Vergani F, Fernandez-Miranda JC. Meninges and ventricular system. In: Standring S, editor. Gray's anatomy: the anatomic basis of clinical practice. 42nd edition. Philadelphia: Elsevier; 2020. p. 398–414.e2.

17. San Millán Ruíz D, Gailloud P, Rüfenacht DA, et al. The craniocervical venous system in relation to cerebral venous drainage. AJNR Am J Neuroradiol 2002; 23(9):1500–8.

18. Shimizu S. Epidural" vertebral venous plexus. AJNR Am J Neuroradiol 2006;27(1):7. author reply 7.

19. Bailey MA, Holroyd HR, Patel JV, et al. The right vertebral artery arising as a branch of the right internal carotid artery: report of a rare case. Surg Radiol Anat 2009;31(10):819–21.

20. Littooy FN, Baker WH, Field TC, et al. Anomalous branches of the cervical internal carotid artery: two cases of clinical importance. J Vasc Surg 1988; 8(5):634–7.

21. Quint DJ, Boulos RS, Spera TD. Congenital absence of the cervical and petrous internal carotid artery with intercavernous anastomosis. AJNR Am J Neuroradiol 1989;10(2):435–9.

22. Gailloud P, Carpenter J, Heck DV, et al. Pseudofenestration of the cervical internal carotid artery: a pathologic process that simulates an anatomic variant. AJNR Am J Neuroradiol 2004;25(3):421–4.

23. Gumus T, Onal B, Ilgit ET. Bilateral persistence of type 1 proatlantal arteries: report of a case and review of the literature. AJNR Am J Neuroradiol 2004;25(9):1622–4.

24. Lukins DE, Pilati S, Escott EJ. The moving carotid artery: a retrospective review of the retropharyngeal carotid artery and the incidence of positional changes on serial studies. AJNR Am J Neuroradiol 2016;37(2):336–41.

25. Koreckij J, Alvi H, Gibly R, et al. Incidence and risk factors of the retropharyngeal carotid artery on cervical magnetic resonance imaging. Spine (Phila Pa 1976) 2013;38(2):E109–12.

26. Sacco S, Totaro R, Baldassarre M, et al. Morphological variations of the internal carotid artery: prevalence, characteristics and association with cerebrovascular disease. Int J Angiol 2007;16(2):59–61.

27. Lo WW, Solti-Bohman LG, McElveen JT Jr. Aberrant carotid artery: radiologic diagnosis with emphasis on high-resolution computed tomography. Radiographics 1985;5(6):985–93.

28. Glastonbury CM, Harnsberger HR, Hudgins PA, et al. Lateralized petrous internal carotid artery: imaging features and distinction from the aberrant internal carotid artery. Neuroradiology 2012;54(9):1007–13.

29. Luh GY, Dean BL, Tomsick TA, et al. The persistent fetal carotid-vertebrobasilar anastomoses. AJR Am J Roentgenol 1999;172(5):1427–32.

30. Pereira Filho Ade A, Gobbato PL, Pereira Filho Gde A, et al. Intracranial intrasellar kissing carotid arteries: case report. Arq Neuropsiquiatr 2007; 65(2A):355–7.

31. Cetin I, Varan B, Orün UA, et al. Common trunks of the subclavian and the vertebral arteries: presentation of a new aortic arch anomaly. Ann Vasc Surg 2009;23(1):142–3.

32. Moshayedi P, Walker GB, Tavakoli S, et al. Dual origin of the right vertebral artery from the right common carotid and aberrant right subclavian arteries. J Clin Neurosci 2018;53:258–60.

33. Kim MS. Duplicated vertebral artery: literature review and clinical significance. J Korean Neurosurg Soc 2018;61(1):28–34.

34. Eskander MS, Drew JM, Aubin ME, et al. Vertebral artery anatomy: a review of two hundred fifty magnetic resonance imaging scans. Spine (Phila Pa 1976) 2010;35(23):2035–40.

35. Provenzale JM, Sarikaya B, Hacein-Bey L, et al. Causes of misinterpretation of cross-sectional imaging studies for dissection of the craniocervical arteries. AJR Am J Roentgenol 2011;196(1):45–52.

36. Kulyk C, Voltan C, Simonetto M, et al. Vertebral artery hypoplasia: an innocent lamb or a disguise? J Neurol 2018;265(10):2346–52.

37. Zivelonghi C, Emiliani A, Micheletti N, et al. Vertebral artery fenestration mimicking acute dissection. Ann Neurol 2020;88(2):235–6.

38. Atmaca S, Elmali M, Kucuk H. High and dehiscent jugular bulb: clear and present danger during middle ear surgery. Surg Radiol Anat 2014;36(4):369–74.

39. Kupfer RA, Hoesli RC, Green GE, et al. The relationship between jugular bulb-vestibular aqueduct dehiscence and hearing loss in pediatric patients. Otolaryngol Head Neck Surg 2012;146(3):473–7.

40. Raghuram K, Curé JK, Harnsberger HR. Condylar jugular diverticulum. J Comput Assist Tomogr 2009;33(2):309–11.

41. Bilgen C, Kirazli T, Ogut F, et al. Jugular bulb diverticula: clinical and radiologic aspects. Otolaryngol Head Neck Surg 2003;128(3):382–6.

42. Lim CL, Keshava SN, Lea M. Anatomical variations of the internal jugular veins and their relationship to the carotid arteries: a CT evaluation. Australas Radiol 2006;50(4):314–8.

43. Asouhidou I, Natsis K, Asteri T, et al. Anatomical variation of left internal jugular vein: clinical

significance for an anaesthesiologist. Eur J Anaesthesiol 2008;25(4):314–8.

44. Jayaraman MV, Boxerman JL, Davis LM, et al. Incidence of extrinsic compression of the internal jugular vein in unselected patients undergoing CT angiography. AJNR Am J Neuroradiol 2012;33(7):1247–50.

45. McKinney AM. Miscellaneous cervical venous variants. In: Atlas of normal imaging variations of the brain, skull, and craniocervical vasculature. Cham: Springer; 2017. p. 1023–34.

46. Towbin AJ, Kanal E. A review of two cases of fenestrated internal jugular veins as seen by CT angiography. AJNR Am J Neuroradiol 2004;25(8):1433–4.

47. Comert E, Comert A. External jugular vein duplication. J Craniofac Surg 2009;20(6):2173–4.

48. Mahalingam HV, Mani SE, Patel B, et al. Imaging spectrum of cavernous sinus lesions with histopathologic correlation. Radiographics 2019;39(3):795–819.

49. Alcaide-Leon P, López-Rueda A, Coblentz A, et al. Prominent inferior intercavernous sinus on sagittal T1-weighted images: a sign of intracranial hypotension. AJR Am J Roentgenol 2016;206(4):817–22.

50. McKinney AM. Emissary veins, vascular-containing foramina, and vascular depressions of the skull. In: Atlas of normal imaging variations of the brain, skull, and craniocervical vasculature. Cham: Springer; 2017. p. 859–85.

51. Bunch PM, Hughes RT, White EP, et al. The pharyngolaryngeal venous plexus: a potential pitfall in surveillance imaging of the neck. AJNR Am J Neuroradiol 2021;42(5):938–44.

52. Nguyen RP, Shah LM, Quigley EP, et al. Carotid body detection on CT angiography. AJNR Am J Neuroradiol 2011;32(6):1096–9.

53. Ward PJ. Mediastinum. In: Standring S, editor. Gray's anatomy: the anatomic basis of clinical practice. 42nd edition. Philadelphia: Elsevier; 2020. p. 1047–67.e1.

54. Liu ME, Branstetter BF 4th, Whetstone J, et al. Normal CT appearance of the distal thoracic duct. AJR Am J Roentgenol 2006;187(6):1615–20.

Parathyroid Computed Tomography
Pearls, Pitfalls, and Our Approach

Hillary R. Kelly, MD[a],*, Paul M. Bunch, MD[b]

KEYWORDS

- Hyperparathyroidism • 4D CT • Parathyroid ultrasound • Parathyroid adenoma

KEY POINTS

- Parathyroid imaging is for localization, not diagnosis. The radiologist's role is to anatomically map candidate parathyroid lesions in order to facilitate successful operative cure of hyperparathyroidism.
- Multiphase parathyroid computed tomography (CT) (4-dimensional [4D] CT) has emerged as a favored modality for preoperative parathyroid imaging, both as a first-line approach and as a problem-solving tool in difficult and reoperative cases.
- Ultrasound is low-cost, widely available, avoids ionizing radiation, and can effectively complement 4D CT to increase parathyroid lesion preoperative localization confidence.
- Parathyroid imaging is most successful when performed as a multidisciplinary, multimodality collaboration, integrating clinical and surgical information with all available imaging studies to inform the preoperative localization. It is imperative to subsequently correlate the ultimate operative and pathologic results with the original localization for continual practice improvement.

INTRODUCTION

Hyperparathyroidism is a common endocrine disorder caused by abnormal function of one or more parathyroid glands, resulting in inappropriate secretion of excess parathyroid hormone. Imaging has no role in the diagnosis of hyperparathyroidism, which is made by serum biochemical testing.[1,2] Surgery is the only curative option. Primarily used in patients with primary hyperparathyroidism, surgery is less commonly performed in cases of secondary or tertiary hyperparathyroidism resistant to medical management.[1,2] Thorough reviews of parathyroid anatomy, embryology, imaging localization options, and parathyroid surgery are available in the August 2021 issue of this journal (see Sara B. Strauss's article, "Parathyroid Imaging: Four-dimensional Computed Tomography, Sestamibi, and Ultrasonography" and Aditya S. Shirali's article, "Parathyroid Surgery: What the Radiologist Needs to Know," in that issue).[3,4] This article focuses on our experience with multiphase parathyroid computed tomography (CT), or 4-dimensional CT (4D CT), as a primary imaging modality for preoperative localization in patients with primary hyperparathyroidism, including pearls and pitfalls, how to problem-solve in difficult cases, and the use of ultrasonography as a complementary and supportive modality.

IMAGING TECHNIQUE
Multiphase Parathyroid Computed Tomography

Parathyroid CT (also known as "4D CT") consists of multiphase CT of the neck acquired from the maxilla to the carina with multiplanar

a Department of Radiology, Massachusetts General Hospital, Massachusetts Eye and Ear and Harvard Medical School, 55 Fruit Street, Boston, MA 02114, USA; b Department of Radiology, Wake Forest School of Medicine, Medical Center Boulevard, Winston Salem, NC 27157, USA
* Corresponding author.
E-mail address: hillary.kelly@mgh.harvard.edu

Neuroimag Clin N Am 32 (2022) 413–431
https://doi.org/10.1016/j.nic.2022.01.006
1052-5149/22/© 2022 Elsevier Inc. All rights reserved.

Box 1
Parathyroid computed tomography: imaging protocols

- Position: supine; head first in scanner; arms down and extended caudally by use of manufacturer-supplied straps
- Scan coverage: maxilla to carina for all phases (noncontrast, enhanced, arterial, and venous)
- Iodinated contrast material administration: 100 mL (350–370 mg iodine/mL, depending on the institution) injected at 4 mL/s, followed by 40 mL saline flush
  - Arterial phase: 30 sec after the start of the injection
  - Venous phase: 30 sec after the completion of the arterial phase
- Detector coverage: 40 mm
- Slice thickness: 1.25 mm
- Interval: 1 mm
- Tube voltage: 140 kVp
- Tube current (automatic modulation): 180 to 300 mA (min to max)
- Noise index: 10
- Pitch: 1.375
- Rotation time: 1 sec
- Display field of view (DFOV): 25 cm
- Images reconstructed:
  - 1.25 mm (all phases)
  - 2.5 mm coronal, 2.5 mm sagittal (arterial)
- CTDIvol (per phase): 19 to 24 mGy (32-cm phantom)

reconstructions. The fourth dimension refers to the change in attenuation over time.[5] Most protocols include a noncontrast phase followed by arterial and venous phases. There has been extensive debate in the literature over the optimum number of phases[6–15]; however, in our experience we have found greatest success with a 3-phase protocol (**Box 1**).

Training CT technologists in best image acquisition practices minimizes inconsistent or suboptimal image quality. Patients should be scanned in the arms-down position. We use manufacturer-supplied straps to lower the arms as much as tolerated, which decreases artifacts from the shoulders and clavicles (**Figs. 1A–C**). A right-sided injection is preferred to minimize streak artifact in the superior mediastinum and base of the neck from dense iodinated contrast in the left

brachiocephalic vein (**Fig. 1D**). Patients are coached to expect flushing and warmth with the iodinated contrast bolus and repeatedly reminded to avoid coughing or swallowing during image acquisition (**Fig. 2**).[16]

When localizing abnormal parathyroid glands using parathyroid CT, the differential diagnosis is limited—namely, parathyroid gland, thyroid nodule or exophytic thyroid tissue, lymph node, and blood vessel. However, parathyroid lesions are often small with variable location and number. As such, high-quality CT images are critical. Furthermore, the population undergoing parathyroid CT is notably different from the general radiology patient population in that (1) pretest probability of disease is 100%, (2) the parathyroid CT results often substantially affect the operative plan and its likelihood of success, and (3) almost all patients will be cured by surgery and therefore will never require parathyroid CT again in their lifetime (as opposed to lung cancer screening CT, for example). The average age of primary hyperparathyroidism disease onset is the fifth to sixth decades of life and estimates of parathyroid CT lifetime attributable cancer risk remain very low.[17] Considering these factors, we believe it is wholly appropriate for the parathyroid CT acquisition technique to use parameters that result in a higher patient radiation exposure (eg, 19–24 mGy CTDIvol per phase[18]) than routine neck CT to maximize likelihood of a confident, accurate localization that will lead to a curative surgery and minimize the risk of a missed parathyroid lesion resulting from inadequate image quality.

Some investigators advocate omitting the noncontrast phase.[7,8,12–15] However, we find the noncontrast phase to be indispensable and caution that excluding it risks a substantial negative impact on interpretation performance. In fact, it is estimated that up to 25% of parathyroid lesions could be missed without the noncontrast CT phase.[6] In addition, the noncontrast phase decreases false-positive candidate lesions by allowing for accurate characterization of exophytic thyroid tissue (eg, Zuckerkandl tubercle) based on the presence of intrinsic hyperattenuating iodine.

One interpretation challenge is that thyroid disease and primary hyperparathyroidism commonly coexist,[19,20] and diminished thyroid iodine content from chronic thyroid disease (eg, Hashimoto disease) results in abnormal hypoattenuation of the thyroid gland (**Fig. 3**). In these patients, using the noncontrast images to differentiate parathyroid lesions from the thyroid gland is more difficult. Dual-energy parathyroid CT (**Box 2**) has the potential to overcome this limitation in patients with

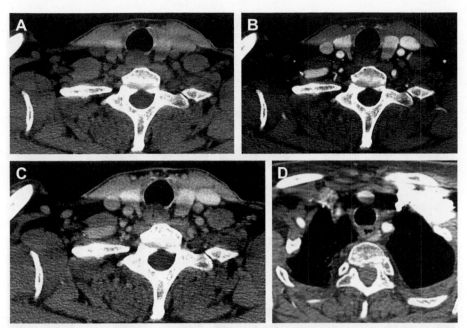

Fig. 1. Artifacts in parathyroid CT. Axial multiphase parathyroid CT images in noncontrast (*A*), arterial phase (*B*) and venous phase (*C*) show streak artifact from the clavicles, resulting in an artifactual band of hypoattenuation through the posterior right and left thyroid lobes on all phases. This artifact could potentially falsely suggest a lesion hypoattenuating to the thyroid parenchyma on the noncontrast or venous phases or could obscure an arterially enhancing candidate parathyroid lesion in this region on the arterial phase. (*D*) Axial postcontrast CT demonstrates a dense iodinated contrast bolus in the left subclavian and brachiocephalic veins, resulting in dark streak artifact across the anterior aspect of the trachea. A candidate parathyroid lesion in the pretracheal space along the lower pole of either thyroid lobe would not be detectable on this study.

diminished thyroid iodine content by using non-contrast 40 keV virtual monoenergetic images to disproportionately increase the Hounsfield unit attenuation and contrast-to-noise ratio of thyroid relative to parathyroid lesions (**Fig. 4**).[16] This disproportionate increase in both attenuation and contrast-to-noise ratio occurs because the CT attenuation of an element is maximal at or slightly greater than the element's K-edge (33.2 keV for iodine).[21,22]

Dual-energy postprocessing can also be used to generate virtual noncontrast images with the potential to decrease patient radiation dose by eliminating the standard noncontrast phase[12,23]; however, we caution against this approach because intrinsic thyroid iodine is also masked, thereby eliminating the utility of the true noncontrast phase for differentiating parathyroid lesions from thyroid tissue by thyroid iodine content.

Parathyroid Ultrasound

Ultrasound is a common first-line modality for parathyroid imaging. Before the advent of multiphase parathyroid CT, the combination of ultrasound and parathyroid scintigraphy was considered standard of care for preoperative parathyroid localization.[5,10] Ultrasound has a sensitivity of approximately 80% in primary hyperparathyroidism caused by a single parathyroid adenoma,[24] but only 15% to 35% in multigland disease.[25]

In our experience, ultrasound is an effective complementary imaging modality that increases confidence in localizing parathyroid lesions when used in concordance with multiphase parathyroid CT. Advantages of ultrasound include low cost, lack of ionizing radiation, widespread availability, excellent anatomic resolution, ability to assess for concurrent thyroid neoplasms, and potential for image-guided fine-needle aspiration sampling of candidate parathyroid lesions.[26] Ultrasound is often used by surgeons in their offices or in the operating room,[27,28] which can streamline care and decrease costs. Because in-office and intraoperative images are usually not captured or available for subsequent comparison, we prefer to perform ultrasound in the same imaging appointment as multiphase 4D CT and interpret the imaging studies simultaneously, often characterizing

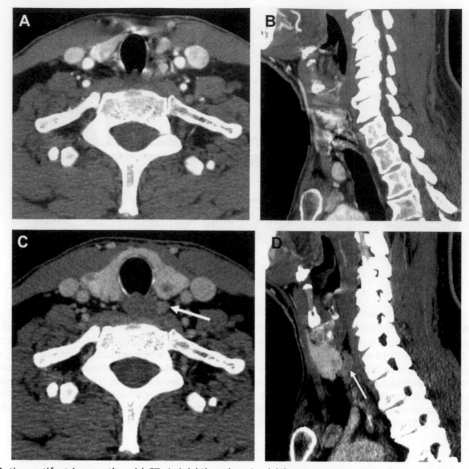

Fig. 2. Motion artifact in parathyroid CT. Axial (A) and sagittal (B) postcontrast CT in the arterial phase demonstrates motion artifact related to coughing obscuring and distorting the thyroid gland and adjacent structures. (C, D) A left superior parathyroid adenoma (arrows) is seen as a nodule hypoattenuating to the adjacent thyroid gland on the axial (C) and sagittal (D) venous phase postcontrast CT images, which were not degraded by motion.

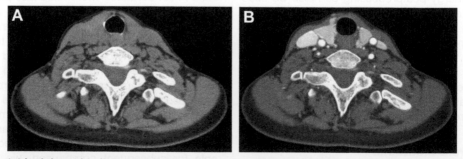

Fig. 3. Diminished thyroid iodine content. The intrinsic thyroid iodine content is so low in this case that the thyroid cannot be distinguished from the adjacent musculature or unenhanced vascular structures on the axial noncontrast (A) parathyroid CT image. The boundaries between the thyroid gland and the adjacent structures are only apparent after the administration of intravenous contrast (B).

Box 2
Dual-energy parathyroid computed tomography: imaging protocols

- Position: supine; head first in scanner; arms down and extended caudally by use of manufacturer supplied straps
- Scan coverage: maxilla to carina for all phases (noncontrast, enhanced, arterial, and venous)
- Iodinated contrast material administration: 100 mL (350–370 mg iodine/mL, depending on the institution) injected at 4 mL/s, followed by 40 mL saline flush
  - Arterial phase: 30 sec after the start of the injection
  - Venous phase: 30 sec after the completion of the arterial phase
- Detector coverage: 40 mm
- Helical thickness: 2.5 mm
- Interval: 2.5 mm
- Tube voltage: 80/140 kVp (fast-kVp switching)
- Tube current (automatic modulation): 250 to 445 mA (min to max)
- Pitch: 0.516:1
- Rotation time: 0.5 sec
- Display field of view (DFOV): 25 cm
- Images reconstructed:
  - 0.63 mm axial (all phases)
  - 2 mm coronal (noncontrast and arterial)
  - 2 mm sagittal (arterial)
- Reconstruction method: ASiR-V 20%
- Convolution kernel: "Standard"
- CTDIvol (per phase): 11 to 24 mGy (32-cm phantom)

lesions as thyroid or parathyroid based on both CT and ultrasound features. Multimodality concordance also increases the likelihood that surgeons will offer minimally invasive parathyroidectomy or repeat surgical exploration in cases of persistent or recurrent hyperparathyroidism.

IMAGING INTERPRETATION AND REPORTING
Search Pattern and Search Strategy

Although important for interpreting all imaging examinations, an effective search pattern and successful search strategy are particularly important in parathyroid imaging, given the 100% pretest probability of hyperparathyroidism and the desire for confident and accurate localization to facilitate operative cure. Knowledge of where to find diseased parathyroid glands informs the search pattern, and an understanding of parathyroid lesion imaging characteristics informs the strategy.

Although normal superior parathyroid glands are most commonly found within 1 cm of the junction of the cricoid and thyroid cartilages,[1] adenomatous or otherwise enlarged superior glands have a tendency to descend posteriorly and inferiorly presumably due to gravity into the tracheoesophageal groove[29,30] or even more posteriorly into a retropharyngeal, retrolaryngeal, or retroesophageal (Fig. 5) position.[1] This change in position of an enlarged gland from increased mass is known as "acquired ectopia" or "acquired migration," which can also affect the inferior glands. Rarely (<1%), a superior gland will be located directly adjacent to the carotid artery within the carotid sheath (Fig. 6), within the thyroid parenchyma (Fig. 7), or lateral to the carotid in the scalene fat pad.[1] Therefore, we initially search for superior glands along the posterior aspects of the upper thyroid lobes and then expand our search for the superior glands to a wider area along the plane of and posterior to the tracheoesophageal groove, including retroesophageal and retropharyngeal locations between the suprahyoid neck and superior mediastinum (Fig. 8).

Approximately half of normal inferior parathyroid glands are found within 1 cm posterior, inferior, or lateral to the lower pole of the thyroid.[1] However, ectopic inferior parathyroid glands can be found anywhere from the angle of the mandible to the level of the lower thymus and pericardium in the anterior mediastinum. In searching for the inferior glands, we first focus along all margins of the thyroid gland anterior to the tracheoesophageal groove, with particular attention to the inferior aspects of the lower poles (Fig. 9). If no high-confidence candidate lesion has been identified after a thorough search of the axial images, scrutiny of the coronal images along the inferior aspects of the thyroid lobes (Fig. 10) may be fruitful. We then expand the search into the lower neck and anterior mediastinum in areas most likely to contain ectopic or inferiorly migrated inferior parathyroid glands (Fig. 11). When acquired migration of inferior parathyroid glands occurs, the path of descent is often through the thyrothymic ligament (thymic remnant) immediately posterior to the strap muscles to reach the anterior mediastinum and thymus (Fig. 12). Rarely (<1%) an inferior gland will be located within the carotid sheath (Fig. 13) or within the thyroid parenchyma.[1]

Parathyroid lesions will always be hypoattenuating relative to the normal thyroid parenchyma on

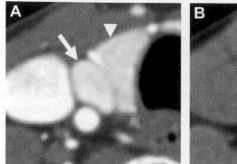
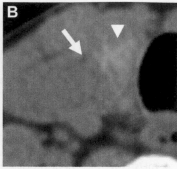
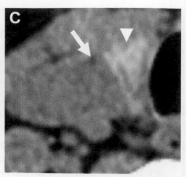

Fig. 4. Discriminating parathyroid lesions from thyroid gland using dual-energy CT 40 keV virtual monoenergetic images. Axial parathyroid CT arterial phase image (*A*) demonstrates a right inferior parathyroid adenoma (*arrow, A*) along the lateral aspect of the right thyroid lobe. Because the adenoma abuts and is isoattenuating to the adjacent thyroid gland (*arrowhead, A*), it could be easily overlooked on the arterial phase. Careful examination of the standard (70 keV) dual-energy CT noncontrast image (*B*) shows the adenoma (*arrow, B*) to be hypoattenuating relative to the adjacent iodine-containing thyroid gland (*arrowhead, B*). The 40 keV dual-energy CT noncontrast image (*C*) accentuates the difference in attenuation between the thyroid gland and adjacent parathyroid adenoma relative to the standard noncontrast image. The window (400 HU) and level (40 HU) settings are identical in both noncontrast images (*B, C*).

the noncontrast phase. However, parathyroid lesions will commonly abut and be nearly isoattenuating to the thyroid gland on one or both of the contrast-enhanced CT phases (**Fig. 14**). One strategy to avoid overlooking such lesions is to review the noncontrast phase first, paying special attention to the periphery of the thyroid gland and making a mental checklist of hypoattenuating (ie, "nonthyroid") soft tissue nodules to be scrutinized as candidate parathyroid lesions on the arterial and venous phases.

Regardless of the search pattern used, it is important to follow the search through to completion at each location to minimize the risk of missing

supernumerary parathyroid tissue, even when a high-confidence candidate lesion is identified early in the search.

Image Interpretation and Reporting

Once the search has been completed, the radiologist must then decide which findings to describe as candidate parathyroid lesions. The classic parathyroid adenoma enhancement pattern of hyperattenuating relative to thyroid on the arterial phase and hypoattenuating or "washout" on the venous phase is well described. However, this classic enhancement pattern is observed in only

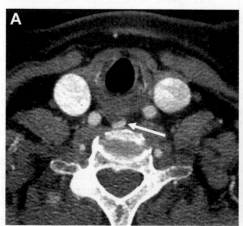
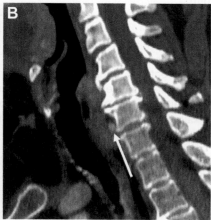

Fig. 5. Axial (*A*) and sagittal (*B*) parathyroid CT arterial phase images demonstrate a right superior parathyroid adenoma (*arrows*) in a retroesophageal location, closely abutting the prevertebral fascia. Such posterior lesions cannot be identified by ultrasound due to depth and shadowing from the airway and laryngeal or tracheal cartilages.

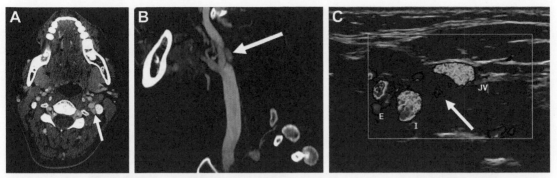

Fig. 6. Ectopic left superior parathyroid within the carotid sheath. Axial (*A*) and sagittal (*B*) parathyroid CT arterial phase images demonstrate an enhancing lesion (*arrows, A* and *B*) closely abutting the left internal carotid artery and left internal jugular vein. Transverse Doppler image (*C*) from an ultrasound performed at the same imaging appointment confirmed a hypoechoic and hypervascular lesion (*arrow, C*) situated between the left internal carotid artery (I) and left internal jugular vein (JV) at the level of the carotid bifurcation (E = left external carotid artery).

20% of parathyroid adenomas.[6] Therefore, reliance on enhancement patterns in deciding parathyroid lesion likelihood is a pitfall when interpreting parathyroid CT. Moreover, cystic foci, fat deposition, or calcification may also be observed.[18] Central low attenuation representing cystic degeneration, old hemorrhage, or fibrosis can be a clue that a lesion is parathyroid in origin.[31,32] However, cases of very large predominantly cystic (**Fig. 15**) or completely cystic parathyroid lesions can mimic other pathology such as thymic (**Fig. 16**) or foregut duplication cysts. Fine-needle aspiration sampling for parathyroid hormone content may be helpful in such instances (see **Fig. 16**).

Given the highly variable appearance of parathyroid lesions and the 100% pretest probability of abnormal parathyroid gland, we advocate describing any structure as a candidate parathyroid lesion that is not clearly thyroid, lymph node, or vascular. Unlike parathyroid lesions, normal thyroid tissue exhibits hyperattenuation on the noncontrast CT phase due to the intrinsic iodine content. A fatty hilum and progressive enhancement pattern (hyperattenuating on the venous phase relative to the arterial phase) are characteristic of lymph nodes; however, a potentially more practical method of assessment is to compare the candidate in question with several jugular chain lymph nodes on both contrast-enhanced

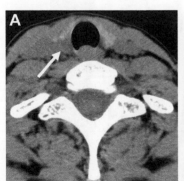
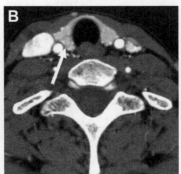
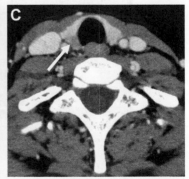

Fig. 7. Intrathyroidal right superior parathyroid adenoma. This patient was status post removal of a right inferior parathyroid adenoma along the lower pole of the right thyroid lobe but had persistent hypercalcemia and elevated parathyroid hormone. Axial noncontrast (*A*), arterial (*B*), and venous (*C*) parathyroid CT images demonstrate a lesion that was nearly indistinguishable from the thyroid parenchyma on the arterial phase (*arrow, B*) but was hypoattenuating relative to the thyroid gland on the noncontrast images (*arrow, A*) and demonstrated washout of contrast on the venous phase (*arrow, C*). During the repeat surgery, the thyroid capsule was opened and explored based on this multiphase parathyroid CT study, and an intrathyroidal parathyroid adenoma was discovered and pathologically confirmed.

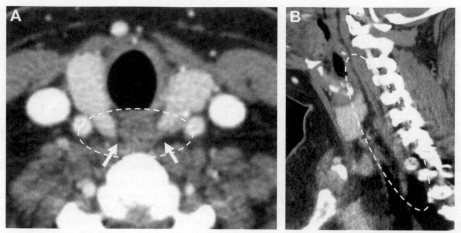

Fig. 8. Search areas for diseased superior parathyroid glands. Axial (A) and sagittal (B) parathyroid CT arterial phase images demonstrate the typical location of superior parathyroid glands along the posterior aspect of the upper thyroid lobes (arrows). Superior parathyroid lesions may also be found within and posterior to the tracheoesophageal grooves (including the paraesophageal, retroesophageal, and retropharyngeal locations) from the hyoid to the superior mediastinum (dashed ovals, A and B).

phases. If the enhancement of the candidate lesion seems identical to the jugular chain lymph nodes on both phases, we typically conclude that the candidate is more likely a lymph node than a parathyroid lesion. Otherwise, we describe the finding as a candidate parathyroid lesion. When present, a polar vessel increases confidence that a lesion is of parathyroid origin (as opposed to the hilar blood supply of a lymph node).[33]

Reporting the size and number of candidate parathyroid lesions can have important surgical implications. Most cases of primary hyperparathyroidism are the result of a single parathyroid adenoma. However, a substantial minority (up to 30%)[34] are caused by multigland disease. Although minimally invasive parathyroidectomy is often preferred for single adenomas,[35,36] bilateral neck exploration is necessary for multigland disease.[37] Multigland disease is more likely when

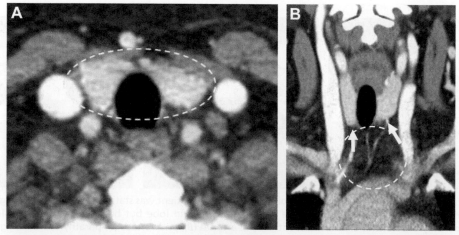

Fig. 9. Initial search areas for diseased inferior parathyroid glands. Axial (A) and coronal (B) parathyroid CT arterial phase images demonstrate the initial search area for inferior parathyroid glands along the posterior, inferior, and lateral aspects of the of the thyroid gland (dashed oval, A) and extending inferiorly toward the mediastinum (dashed oval, B). We often find inferior parathyroid glands just inferior to the lower poles of the thyroid gland (arrows, B).

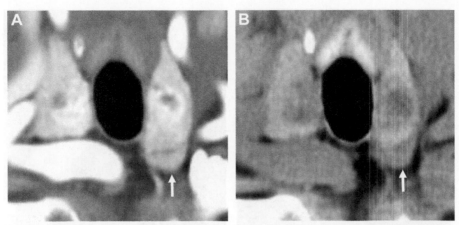

Fig. 10. Coronal reformats facilitate identification of difficult-to-find inferior parathyroid lesions. Coronal arterial phase (*A*) and noncontrast phase (*B*) images demonstrate a left inferior parathyroid adenoma (*arrows*) along the inferior margin of the left thyroid lobe. This lesion was not appreciated to be separate from the thyroid gland on review of axial images, likely because of volume averaging effects and near isoattenuation to the thyroid gland on the arterial phase. Coronal reformats showed to greater advantage both the plane between the parathyroid adenoma and the inferior margin of the left thyroid lobe as well as the hypodensity of the adenoma relative to the iodine-containing thyroid gland on the noncontrast phase.

there are (1) multiple candidate parathyroid lesions, (2) no identifiable parathyroid lesions, or (3) the largest candidate lesion measures less than 7 mm in maximum dimension.[38] Satisfaction of search is always a potential pitfall in parathyroid imaging. Although larger lesions favor single gland disease, multigland disease remains a possibility, and any coinciding candidate lesions should also be described (**Fig. 17**). It is far better to alert the surgeon to the presence and exact location of

lower confidence additional lesions that may or may not require removal to achieve biochemical cure, as neglecting to describe a lesion that the surgeon must ultimately locate and remove deprives both the patient and the surgeon of the important benefits of preoperative imaging. Thus, by meticulously describing the presence and location of all candidate parathyroid lesions and ranking them by level of confidence and size, the radiologist allows the surgeon to develop a

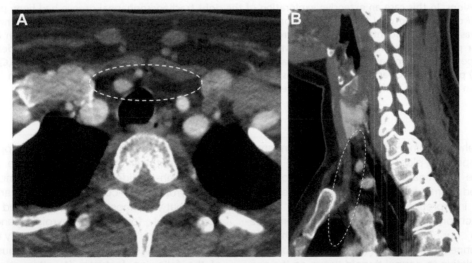

Fig. 11. Search areas for inferiorly migrated inferior parathyroid lesions. Axial (*A*) and sagittal (*B*) parathyroid CT images demonstrate the areas to search along the expected course of the thyroid remnant (thyrothymic ligament) immediately deep to the strap muscles and extending into the anterior mediastinum (*ovals, A* and *B*).

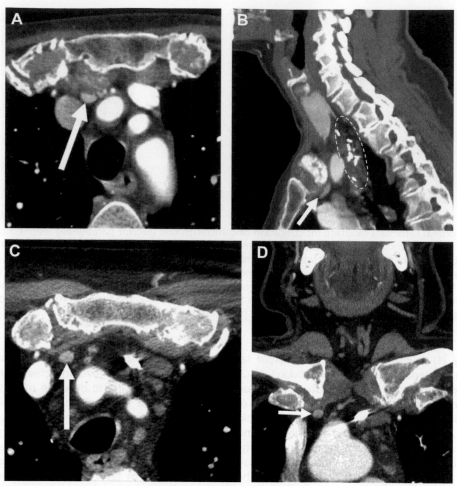

Fig. 12. Migration of inferior parathyroid adenomas. Axial (*A*) and sagittal (*B*) parathyroid CT arterial phase images demonstrate an "inferiorly descended" or migrated right inferior parathyroid adenoma (*arrows*) posterior and inferior to the right sternoclavicular joint (so-called acquired ectopia). It is important to scrutinize the regions immediately posterior to the strap muscles, sternum, and clavicular heads and to describe the anterior location of these lesions. In this case an extensive exploration of the right tracheoesophageal groove had been performed (*surgical clips, dashed oval, B*) based on a preoperative parathyroid CT study, in which a paratracheal lymph node was mistakenly identified as likely corresponding to the site of delayed radiotracer retention described on prior parathyroid scintigraphy (not shown). This inferior parathyroid adenoma was correctly identified at repeat postoperative parathyroid CT images and was ultimately removed at a second surgery. Axial (*C*) and coronal (*D*) parathyroid CT arterial phase images demonstrate a similar right inferior parathyroid lesion (*arrows, C* and *D*) in a different patient, posterior to the right sternoclavicular joint.

comprehensive, individualized, and contingency-laden operative plan.

Some investigators have advocated for standardized terms for reporting confidence levels when interpreting parathyroid CT.[39,40] The approach proposed in the second reference describes our clinical practice in which high-confidence lesions exhibit (1) definite hypoattenuation relative to normal thyroid tissue on the noncontrast phase, (2) enhancement characteristics definitively different from lymph nodes on the

contrast-enhanced phases, and (3) an appearance inconsistent with a blood vessel. We describe these high-confidence lesions as "most likely parathyroid." Low-confidence lesions are candidates that we choose to describe based on location typical for a parathyroid gland while acknowledging that the lesion is unlikely to represent an enlarged parathyroid gland because of one of the following features: (1) attenuation nearly matching the normal thyroid gland on the noncontrast phase (favoring exophytic thyroid tissue), (2)

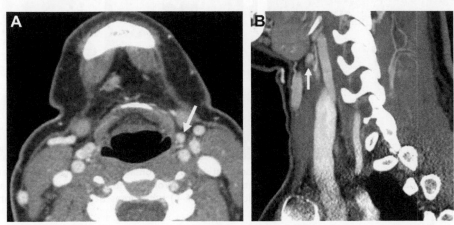

Fig. 13. Undescended left inferior parathyroid. This patient had persistent hyperparathyroidism after undergoing a 7-hour bilateral neck exploration including a left hemithyroidectomy and partial thymectomy, as the left inferior parathyroid could not be found. Postoperative parathyroid CT arterial phase images in axial (*A*) and sagittal (*B*) planes demonstrate a parathyroid adenoma (*arrows*) at the level of the pyriform sinus immediately anterior to the left common carotid artery. At repeat surgery this parathyroid was found within the carotid sheath at the apex of ectopic thymic tissue, consistent with an undescended left inferior gland.

enhancement nearly identical to lymph nodes on both contrast-enhanced phases (favoring a lymph node), or (3) linear or tubular morphology rather than a discrete soft tissue nodule (favoring a blood vessel). We describe these low-confidence lesions as "most likely not parathyroid, though parathyroid remains a differential consideration." Intermediate confidence lesions are typically lesions that do not exhibit clear high- or low-confidence features, and we describe these candidates as "either parathyroid or other" (eg, thyroid nodule, lymph node, vascular, as appropriate to the specific candidate lesion).

When describing the locations of parathyroid lesions, we suggest using the tracheoesophageal groove (the sulcus formed by the abutment of the trachea anteriorly and the esophagus posteriorly) as a point of reference. A common pitfall is to attribute superior or inferior gland origin to parathyroid lesions using only their craniocaudal position relative to the thyroid gland. Surgically and anatomically, the relationship of the parathyroid gland to the recurrent laryngeal nerve (approximated on imaging by the plane of the tracheoesophageal groove) more reliably denotes the embryologic origin,[1,29,30] with superior glands positioned posteriorly and inferior glands positioned anteriorly relative to the nerve.[1,18,30] Because of "acquired ectopia," it is not uncommon for a diseased enlarged superior parathyroid adenoma to be located at or below the lower pole of the thyroid gland, often inferior to the

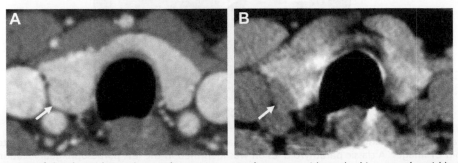

Fig. 14. Scrutiny of the thyroid margins on the noncontrast phase to avoid overlooking parathyroid lesions. Axial arterial phase (*A*) and noncontrast phase (*B*) images demonstrate a right inferior parathyroid adenoma (*arrows*) along the lateral aspect of the right thyroid lobe. On the arterial phase alone, the lesion could be easily overlooked because it abuts and is isoattenuating to the adjacent thyroid gland. However, the lesion is easily identifiable on the noncontrast image because of its hypoattenuation relative to the iodine-containing thyroid gland (see also **Fig. 22**).

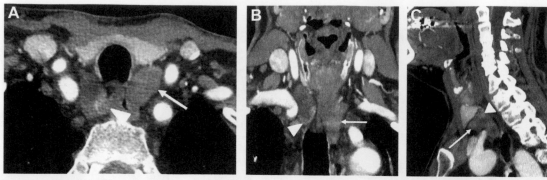

Fig. 15. Large predominantly cystic bilateral superior parathyroid adenomas. Axial (*A*), coronal (*B*), and sagittal (*C*) arterial phase parathyroid CT images demonstrate large parathyroid adenomas in paraesophageal locations bilaterally. These lesions were predominantly cystic (*arrows, A–C*) with areas of solid nodular enhancement peripherally (*arrows, A–C*).

normal inferior parathyroid glands (**Fig. 18**). Incorrect descriptions of embryologic superior parathyroid adenomas located posterior to the tracheoesophageal groove as inferior parathyroid glands based on the location within the inferior neck or superior mediastinum can contribute to failed surgery if the surgeon relies on the radiologist's description to inform the operative approach. If uncertain as to the embryologic origin of a parathyroid lesion, it is also acceptable to simply provide a detailed description of the lesion's location with respect to adjacent structures.

We also use the cricoid cartilage as an additional reference point when describing parathyroid lesions because the cricoid is consistently palpable, visualized in the standard operative field,

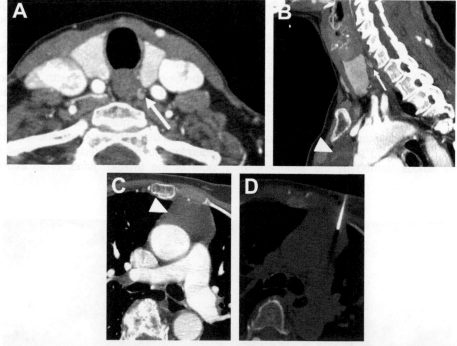

Fig. 16. Large cystic parathyroid adenoma mimicking a thymic cyst. Axial (*A, C*) and sagittal (*B*) arterial phase parathyroid CT images. A classic parathyroid lesion was identified in the left paraesophageal location posterior to the left thyroid upper pole (*arrows, A* and *B*) consistent with a left superior parathyroid adenoma. However, the patient had persistent severe hypercalcemia and elevated parathyroid hormone (PTH) after removal of this pathologically confirmed adenoma. A cystic lesion was also present in the anterior superior mediastinum (*large arrowhead, B* and *C*). A mediastinal MR imaging (not shown) confirmed that this was a completely cystic lesion without solid or enhancing components. CT-guided fine-needle aspiration (*D*) confirmed very high parathyroid hormone content within this lesion, which was subsequently removed by a thoracic surgeon.

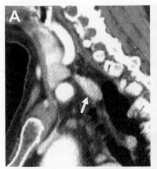
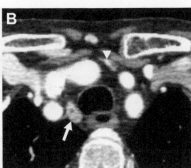
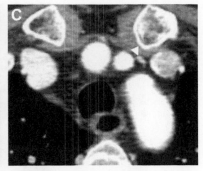

Fig. 17. Avoid satisfaction of search. Sagittal (*A*) and axial (*B, C*) arterial phase images demonstrate a large, "inferiorly descended," right superior parathyroid lesion (*arrows, A* and *B*) measuring 28 mm in long axis (SI). Although large size favors single gland disease, adherence to a thorough search pattern resulted in 2 smaller left inferior parathyroid candidate lesions (*arrowheads B* and *C*) being identified and described. At surgery, removal of all 3 lesions was necessary to achieve biochemical cure.

orients the surgeon to the anatomic midline, and is particularly useful in the reoperative setting. In addition, we look for and describe an aberrant right subclavian artery or far less commonly a right aortic arch with aberrant left subclavian artery because in these situations the recurrent laryngeal nerve ipsilateral to the aberrant subclavian artery exhibits a variant, unpredictable, "nonrecurrent" course, which places the nerve at increased risk of operative injury (up to 13%),[41] especially if the surgeon is not alerted preoperatively.

Problem-Solving Techniques and Skill Development

On occasions when suboptimal image quality (eg, degraded by motion or other artifact) may decrease confidence of interpretation, prior

imaging including the area of interest can be a valuable complement (**Fig. 19**). In fact, there is evidence that abnormal parathyroid glands can be retrospectively identified in most patients with primary hyperparathyroidism with available old imaging, often obtained years before biochemical diagnosis.[42]

Ultrasound can also be a useful problem-solving tool in cases of suboptimal parathyroid CT image quality (**Fig. 20**). Ultrasound is particularly useful in cases with concurrent thyroid pathology[27] (**Fig. 21**). When performed at a concurrent imaging appointment, ultrasound can also help identify lesions on 4D CT that would otherwise be overlooked (**Fig. 22**). Ultrasound-guided fine-needle aspiration can be used to distinguish thyroid nodules from parathyroid adenomas. However, when performing fine-needle aspiration, aspirates

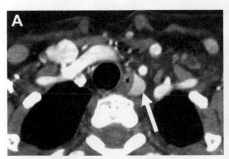
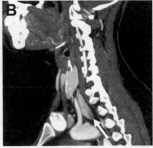
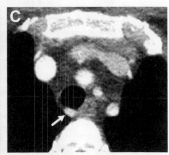

Fig. 18. Acquired migration of superior parathyroid adenomas. Axial (*A*) and sagittal (*B*) parathyroid CT arterial phase images demonstrate an "inferiorly descended" or migrated left superior parathyroid adenoma (*arrows, B* and *C*) in a paraesophageal location, displaced inferiorly and posteriorly (so-called acquired ectopia). Although this gland is located near the lower pole of the left thyroid lobe, the posterior location relative to the expected plane of the recurrent laryngeal nerve identifies this as a superior gland embryologically. (*C*) Axial parathyroid CT arterial phase image in a different patient demonstrates an inferiorly migrated right superior parathyroid gland in the right tracheoesophageal groove at the level of the superior mediastinum, inferior to the plane of the lower poles of the thyroid gland. Diseased superior parathyroid glands can often be found at a level inferior to the thyroid gland.

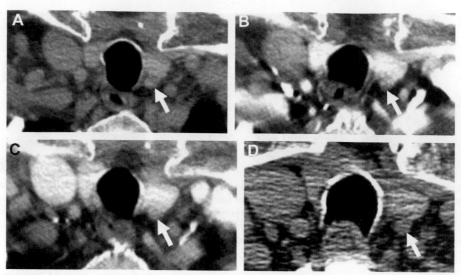

Fig. 19. Value of old imaging. Axial noncontrast (*A*), arterial phase (*B*), and venous phase (*C*) images from a parathyroid CT demonstrate a possible left inferior parathyroid lesion (*arrows*) along the posterior aspect of the left thyroid lobe. However, image artifacts decrease interpretation confidence, particularly of the contrast-enhanced phases. Comparison to a cervical spine CT image (*D*) acquired 7 years before the parathyroid CT increased the radiologist's confidence in the presence of a left inferior parathyroid adenoma in the area of interest (*arrow*), which was confirmed at subsequent surgery.

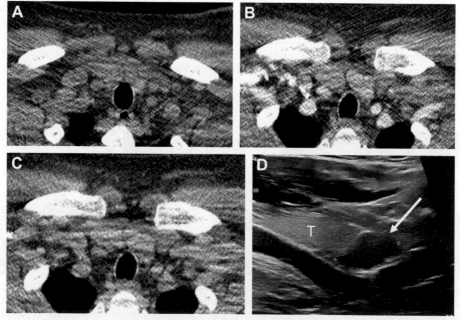

Fig. 20. Parathyroid adenoma at ultrasound. Motion artifact and noise related to patient body habitus resulted in suboptimal image quality on noncontrast (*A*), arterial (*B*), and delayed (*C*) phase axial images at multiphase parathyroid CT. However, an ultrasound was performed immediately following the parathyroid CT at the same imaging appointment, and a parathyroid adenoma was easily identified. Sagittal grayscale image (*D*) demonstrates a left inferior parathyroid adenoma (*arrow, D*) immediately inferior to the lower pole of the left thyroid lobe (*T = thyroid*). Even in retrospect this lesion could not be identified on the same-day parathyroid CT.

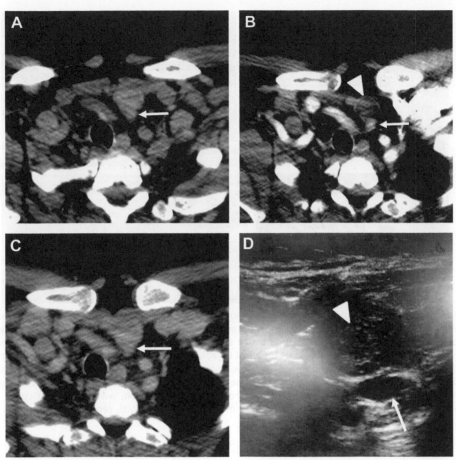

Fig. 21. Parathyroid adenoma at intraop ultrasound. Noncontrast (*A*), arterial (*B*), and delayed (*C*) phase axial parathyroid CT images. A lesion was suspected along the posterior aspect of the left thyroid lobe (*arrow, B*) but confidence was low, as the lesion did not seem hypodense relative to the thyroid gland on the noncontrast phase (*arrow, A*) or on the delayed phase (*arrow, C*) and thyroid tissue posterior to a large thyroid nodule (*arrowhead, B*) was felt to be most likely. However, an ultrasound was performed in the operating room, and a parathyroid adenoma was easily identified. Transverse grayscale image (*D*) demonstrates a left inferior parathyroid adenoma (*arrow, D*) immediately posterior to, but clearly separate from, a left lower pole thyroid nodule (*arrowhead, D*).

should be sent for parathyroid hormone levels, as cytology is less sensitive and parathyroid tissue can be misinterpreted as follicular thyroid lesions (**Fig. 23**) or vice versa.[27,29,43–46]

Parathyroid localization skills are developed and refined with experience and thorough feedback on the accuracy of previous preoperative localizations obtained through correlating imaging findings with operative results. Because parathyroid imaging is typically performed for operative planning, there are ample opportunities for this form of radiologic-pathologic correlation. This process can be made easier by asking your surgeon to route parathyroidectomy operative notes directly to you through your health system's electronic medical record. In addition, practicing as a multidisciplinary team and being involved in discussions with your surgeons both before surgery and while in the operating room can be invaluable, with the potential to both improve radiology interpretation skills via frequent feedback and affect surgical results. Be prepared to receive calls from surgeons seeking real-time help when the most likely candidate lesion identified at imaging is not found at surgery or is shown to represent a mimic such as an exophytic thyroid nodule or lymph node. By providing assistance and imaging expertise in these moments of need, radiologists can build trust with the surgeon and meaningfully contribute to patient care.

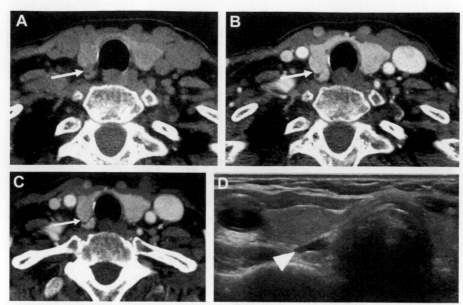

Fig. 22. Right inferior parathyroid identified by ultrasound. Noncontrast (*A*), arterial (*B*), and delayed (*C*) phase axial parathyroid CT images. No lesion was appreciated on initial review of the CT images. However, at ultrasound, transverse grayscale image (*D*) demonstrates a hypoechoic nodule (*arrowhead, D*) situated between normal thyroid tissue along the lower pole of the right thyroid lobe. The lesion at CT is isoattenuating to the thyroid gland on the arterial and delayed images (*arrows, B* and *C*); however, on close scrutiny of the noncontrast images a hypoattenuating nodule (*arrow, A*) can be seen bordered by normal hyperdense thyroid tissue along the right thyroid lower pole. A left superior parathyroid lesion (not shown) was also identified by ultrasound and subsequently at parathyroid CT. This patient had multigland disease with removal of 3.5 glands at surgery.

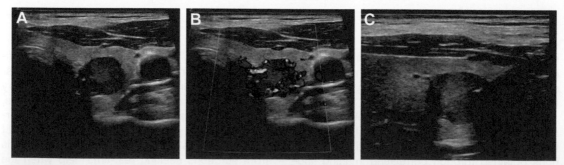

Fig. 23. Parathyroid adenoma mimicking a thyroid nodule. Transverse grayscale (*A*) ultrasound image demonstrates a hypoechoic nodule that seems to be within the midpole of the left thyroid lobe. No candidate parathyroid lesion was identified by ultrasound or parathyroid CT (same patient as **Figs. 1**A–C). Fine-needle aspiration of the finding along the thyroid midpole was performed with report of benign thyroid nodule at cytology. However, marked vascularity of the lesion (color Doppler image *B*) was noted. The surgeon performed an ultrasound-guided fine-needle aspiration (*C*) in the operating room immediately before starting the surgery, and the parathyroid hormone level was reported as 500-fold higher than peripheral blood levels. This parathyroid adenoma was found external to but invaginating into the thyroid capsule.

SUMMARY

Although hyperparathyroidism preoperative imaging algorithms vary, we have found success with parathyroid CT as a primary imaging modality, with ultrasound providing crucial multimodality concordance and serving as a problem-solving tool in difficult cases. When interpreting parathyroid CT, we suggest patterning your search on the knowledge of where normal and diseased parathyroid glands are found. Avoid satisfaction of search and remember that candidate lesion size and number inform the risk of multigland disease and are therefore important to the surgeon. Position relative to the plane of the recurrent laryngeal nerve for which the tracheoesophageal groove is a useful surrogate, rather than superior or inferior location in the neck, determines embryologic origin, and the recurrent laryngeal nerve is at increased risk of operative injury in the setting of an aberrant right subclavian artery. Old imaging can increase interpretation confidence, especially when motion or other artifacts degrade parathyroid CT image quality. Concurrent ultrasound is also useful in cases where parathyroid CT image quality is suboptimal and when performed by an experienced operator, may quickly identify lesions that are indistinguishable from the thyroid gland at CT. Ultrasound is particularly helpful when a candidate lesion is potentially of thyroid versus parathyroid origin and can be used to guide fine-needle aspiration sampling for parathyroid hormone levels in ambiguous cases. By practicing as a member of the multidisciplinary care team and by seeking out and incorporating operative feedback, the parathyroid imager will continue to develop and refine localization skills, build valuable relationships with referring surgeons, and meaningfully participate in the care of hyperparathyroidism patients.

CLINICS CARE POINTS

Parathyroid CT: pearls

- Dual-energy parathyroid CT protocols can facilitate discrimination of parathyroid lesions from thyroid tissue by leveraging 40 keV virtual monochromatic images to disproportionately increase the Hounsfield unit attenuation and contrast-to-noise ratio of the thyroid gland relative to parathyroid lesions.
- Use knowledge of where to find diseased parathyroid glands to inform your search pattern.

- Look for and describe variant subclavian artery anatomy associated with a nonrecurrent laryngeal nerve.
- Review old imaging as well as all other parathyroid localization imaging when available to increase interpretation confidence, especially when the study to be interpreted is compromised by motion or other artifacts.
- Review prior operative reports in cases of recurrent or persistent hyperparathyroidism. Knowing the expected number and laterality of previously removed and presumed remaining glands will inform the imaging search pattern and help structure an informed and valuable report to the surgeon and patient.
- Report the increased likelihood of multigland disease if no identifiable parathyroid lesion is identified, if multiple candidate lesions are seen, or if the largest candidate lesion measures less than 7 mm in maximum dimension.
- Ultrasound is particularly useful in the setting of concurrent thyroid pathology. Suggest fine-needle aspiration sampling for parathyroid hormone levels to differentiate thyroid from parathyroid lesions in indeterminate cases.
- If performing fine-needle aspiration sampling of a candidate parathyroid lesion, aspirate parathyroid hormone levels are more sensitive than cytology for diagnosing parathyroid tissue. It is important to communicate with the cytologist to avoid misinterpretation of parathyroid tissue as follicular thyroid tumors.
- Actively participate as a member of the hyperparathyroidism multidisciplinary care team, seeking out and incorporating operative feedback, to build strong relationships with your referring surgeons and to substantially contribute to patient care.

Parathyroid CT: pitfalls

- Up to 25% of parathyroid lesions can be missed if the noncontrast phase is not acquired or is not scrutinized carefully.
- Premature termination of the search for additional parathyroid lesions when a high-confidence candidate is encountered early in the search (satisfaction of search).
- Overreliance on enhancement patterns or other "classic" parathyroid adenoma features and underappreciation of the highly variable appearance of parathyroid lesions when deciding whether to describe a finding as a candidate parathyroid lesion.
- Incorrectly attributing superior or inferior gland origin to a parathyroid lesion using craniocaudal position relative to the thyroid

gland rather than the plane of the recurrent laryngeal nerve approximated by the tracheoesophageal groove.

- Failure to correlate with ultrasound can result in misinterpretation of a thyroid nodule as a parathyroid lesion and vice versa. Correlation with ultrasound is particularly important in the setting of concurrent thyroid pathology.

DISCLOSURE

H.R. Kelly has served as a Principal Investigator with clinical trial funding provided to her institution by Bayer AG (no personal compensation or salary support).

REFERENCES

1. Cho NL, Doherty GM. Principles in Surgical Management of Primary Hyperparathyroidism. In: Randolph GW, editor. Surgery of the thyroid and parathyroid glands. 3rd ed. Elsevier; 2021. p. 502–16.

2. Shindo M, Lee JA, Lubitz CC, et al. The Changing Landscape of Primary, Secondary, and Tertiary Hyperparathyroidism: Highlights from the American College of Surgeons Panel, "What's New for the Surgeon Caring for Patients with Hyperparathyroidism. J Am Coll Surg 2016;222(6):1240–50.

3. Strauss SB, Roytman M, Phillips CD. Parathyroid Imaging. Neuroimaging Clin N Am 2021;31(3):379–95.

4. Shirali AS, Clemente-Gutierrez U, Perrier ND. Parathyroid Surgery. Neuroimaging Clin N Am 2021; 31(3):397–408.

5. Rodgers SE, Hunter GJ, Hamberg LM, et al. Improved preoperative planning for directed parathyroidectomy with 4-dimensional computed tomography. Surgery 2006;140(6):932–41.

6. Bahl M, Sepahdari AR, Sosa JA, et al. Parathyroid Adenomas and Hyperplasia on Four-dimensional CT Scans: Three Patterns of Enhancement Relative to the Thyroid Gland Justify a Three-Phase Protocol. Radiology 2015;277(2):454–62.

7. Gafton AR, Glastonbury CM, Eastwood JD, et al. Parathyroid Lesions: Characterization with Dual-Phase Arterial and Venous Enhanced CT of the Neck. Am J Neuroradiol 2012;33(5):949–52.

8. Griffith B, Chaudhary H, Mahmood G, et al. Accuracy of 2-Phase Parathyroid CT for the Preoperative Localization of Parathyroid Adenomas in Primary Hyperparathyroidism. Am J Neuroradiol 2015;36(12): 2373–9.

9. Hunter GJ, Ginat DT, Kelly HR, et al. Discriminating Parathyroid Adenoma from Local Mimics by Using Inherent Tissue Attenuation and Vascular Information Obtained with Four-Dimensional CT: Formulation of a Multinomial Logistic Regression Model. Radiology 2014;270(1):168–75.

10. Kelly HR, Hamberg LM, Hunter GJ. 4D-CT for Preoperative Localization of Abnormal Parathyroid Glands in Patients with Hyperparathyroidism: Accuracy and Ability to Stratify Patients by Unilateral versus Bilateral Disease in Surgery-Naïve and Re-Exploration Patients. Am J Neuroradiol 2014;35(1):176–81.

11. Kutler DI, Moquete R, Kazam E, et al. Parathyroid localization with modified 4D-computed tomography and ultrasonography for patients with primary hyperparathyroidism. Laryngoscope 2011;121(6):1219–24.

12. Leiva-Salinas C, Flors L, Durst CR, et al. Detection of parathyroid adenomas using a monophasic dual-energy computed tomography acquisition: diagnostic performance and potential radiation dose reduction. Neuroradiology 2016;58(11):1135–41.

13. Morón F, Delumpa A, Chetta J, et al. Single phase computed tomography is equivalent to dual phase method for localizing hyperfunctioning parathyroid glands in patients with primary hyperparathyroidism: a retrospective review. PoorJ 2017;5:e3506.

14. Noureldine SI, Aygun N, Walden MJ, et al. Multiphase computed tomography for localization of parathyroid disease in patients with primary hyperparathyroidism: How many phases do we really need? Surgery 2014;156(6):1300–7.

15. Raghavan P, Durst CR, Ornan DA, et al. Dynamic CT for Parathyroid Disease: Are Multiple Phases Necessary? Am J Neuroradiol 2014;35(10):1959–64.

16. Bunch PM, Pavlina AA, Lipford ME, et al. Dual-Energy Parathyroid 4D-CT: Improved Discrimination of Parathyroid Lesions from Thyroid Tissue Using Noncontrast 40-keV Virtual Monoenergetic Images. AJNR Am J Neuroradiol 2021;42(11):2001–8.

17. Hoang JK, Reiman RE, Nguyen GB, et al. Lifetime Attributable Risk of Cancer From Radiation Exposure During Parathyroid Imaging: Comparison of 4D CT and Parathyroid Scintigraphy. Am J Roentgenol 2015;204(5):W579–85.

18. Bunch PM, Randolph GW, Brooks JA, et al. Parathyroid 4D CT: What the Surgeon Wants to Know. RadioGraphics 2020;40(5):1383–94.

19. Bentrem DJ, Angelos P, Talamonti MS, et al. Is preoperative investigation of the thyroid justified in patients undergoing parathyroidectomy for hyperparathyroidism? Thyroid Off J Am Thyroid Assoc 2002;12(12):1109–12.

20. Jovanovic MD, Zivaljevic VR, Diklic AD, et al. Surgical treatment of concomitant thyroid and parathyroid disorders: analysis of 4882 cases. Eur Arch Otorhino-laryngol 2017;274(2):997–1004.

21. Potter CA, Sodickson AD. Dual-Energy CT in Emergency Neuroimaging: Added Value and Novel Applications. RadioGraphics 2016;36(7):2186–98.

22. Sachs JR, West TG, Lack CM, et al. How to Incorporate Dual-Energy Computed Tomography Into Your

Neuroradiology Practice: Questions and Answers. J Comput Assist Tomogr 2018;42(6):824–30.

23. Roskies M, Liu X, Hier MP, et al. 3-phase dual-energy CT scan as a feasible salvage imaging modality for the identification of non-localizing parathyroid adenomas: a prospective study. J Otolaryngol - Head Neck Surg 2015;44:44.

24. Cheung K, Wang TS, Farrokhyar F, et al. A Meta-analysis of Preoperative Localization Techniques for Patients with Primary Hyperparathyroidism. Ann Surg Oncol 2012;19(2):577–83.

25. Ruda JM, Hollenbeak CS, Stack BC. A systematic review of the diagnosis and treatment of primary hyperparathyroidism from 1995 to 2003. Otolaryngol–head Neck Surg 2005;132(3):359–72.

26. Bunch PM, Kelly HR. Preoperative Imaging Techniques in Primary Hyperparathyroidism: A Review. JAMA Otolaryngol Neck Surg 2018;144(10):929.

27. Lubitz CC, Duh QY. Guide to Preoperative Parathyroid Localization Testing. In: Randolph GW, editor. Surgery of the thyroid and parathyroid glands. 3rd ed. Elsevier; 2021. p. 494–501.

28. Solorzano CC, Carneiro-Pla DM, Irvin GL. Surgeon-performed ultrasonography as the initial and only localizing study in sporadic primary hyperparathyroidism. J Am Coll Surg 2006;202(1):18–24.

29. Harris R, Ryu H, Vu T, et al. Modern Approach to Surgical Intervention of the Thyroid and Parathyroid Glands. Semin Ultrasound CT MRI 2012;33(2):115–22.

30. Perrier ND, Edeiken B, Nunez R, et al. A Novel Nomenclature to Classify Parathyroid Adenomas. World J Surg 2009;33(3):412–6.

31. Hoang JK, Sung Wk, Bahl M, et al. How to Perform Parathyroid 4D CT: Tips and Traps for Technique and Interpretation. Radiology 2014;270(1):15–24.

32. Carlson D. Parathyroid pathology: hyperparathyroidism and parathyroid tumors. Arch Pathol Lab Med 2010;134(11):1639–44.

33. Bahl M, Muzaffar M, Vij G, et al. Prevalence of the Polar Vessel Sign in Parathyroid Adenomas on the Arterial Phase of 4D CT. Am J Neuroradiol 2014;35(3):578–81.

34. Fraker DL, Harsono H, Lewis R. Minimally Invasive Parathyroidectomy: Benefits and Requirements of Localization, Diagnosis, and Intraoperative PTH Monitoring. Long-Term Results. World J Surg 2009;33(11):2256–65.

35. Minisola S, Cipriani C, Diacinti D, et al. Imaging of the parathyroid glands in primary hyperparathyroidism. Eur J Endocrinol 2016;174(1):D1–8.

36. Parangi S, Pandian TK, Thompson GB. Minimally Invasive Single Gland Parathyroid Exploration. In: Randolph GW, editor. Surgery of the thyroid and parathyroid glands. 3rd ed. Elsevier; 2021. p. 529–36.

37. Siperstein AE, Stephen AE, Milas M. Standard Bilateral Parathyroid Exploration. In: Randolph GW, editor. Surgery of the thyroid and parathyroid glands. 3rd ed. Elsevier; 2021. p. 517–28.

38. Sho S, Yilma M, Yeh MW, et al. Prospective Validation of Two 4D-CT–Based Scoring Systems for Prediction of Multigland Disease in Primary Hyperparathyroidism. Am J Neuroradiol 2016;37(12):2323–7.

39. Malinzak MD, Sosa JA, Hoang J. 4D-CT for Detection of Parathyroid Adenomas and Hyperplasia: State of the Art Imaging. Curr Radiol Rep 2017;5(2):8.

40. Bunch PM, Goyal A, Valenzuela C, et al. Parathyroid 4D CT in Primary Hyperparathyroidism: Exploration of Size Measurements for Identifying Multigland Disease and Guiding Biochemically Successful Parathyroidectomy. Am J Roentgenol 2021. https://doi.org/10.2214/AJR.21.26935.

41. Toniato A, Mazzarotto R, Piotto A, et al. Identification of the nonrecurrent laryngeal nerve during thyroid surgery: 20-year experience. World J Surg 2004;28(7):659–61.

42. Nguyen CJ, Johansson ED, Randle RW, et al. Could parathyroid gland assessment on routine CT prevent Morbidity from Undiagnosed primary hyperparathyroidism? Presented at. Chicago, Illinois: Radiological Society of North America 107th Scientific Assembly and Annual Meeting; 2021.

43. Erbil Y, Salmaslıoğlu A, Kabul E, et al. Use of preoperative parathyroid fine-needle aspiration and parathormone assay in the primary hyperparathyroidism with concomitant thyroid nodules. Am J Surg 2007;193(6):665–71.

44. Abraham D, Sharma PK, Bentz J, et al. Utility of ultrasound-guided fine-needle aspiration of parathyroid adenomas for localization before minimally invasive parathyroidectomy. Endocr Pract 2007;13(4):333–7.

45. Sacks BA, Pallotta JA, Cole A, et al. Diagnosis of parathyroid adenomas: efficacy of measuring parathormone levels in needle aspirates of cervical masses. Am J Roentgenol 1994;163(5):1223–6.

46. Stephen AE, Milas M, Garner CN, et al. Use of surgeon-performed office ultrasound and parathyroid fine needle aspiration for complex parathyroid localization. Surgery 2005;138(6):1143–51.

Pearls, Pitfalls, and Mimics in Pediatric Head and Neck Imaging

Felice D'Arco, MD[a], Lorenzo Ugga, MD, PhD[b],*

KEYWORDS

• Head and neck • Pediatrics • Diagnostic imaging • CT • MR imaging

KEY POINTS

• Most of the neck masses in children have some preference for specific locations, which can help in the differential diagnosis. However, there is substantial overlap in possible localizations of different entities, and some masses in children are typically transpatial.

• Identification of one or more key imaging findings in the right clinical context is often enough to reach a precise radiological diagnosis.

• The modality of choice for the study of head and neck masses in children is MR imaging, with protocols that are different from standard brain imaging.

• Clinical presentation, especially the dermatologic findings, together with the patient's age is important for the correct diagnosis, to guide management and predict evolution over time of the lesion.

• Radiologists need to be familiar with the most recent nomenclature of pediatric head and neck masses.

INTRODUCTION

Children present with a spectrum of head and neck pathologies different from those found in the adult population, with specific image findings and clinical characteristics. As most of these entities determining neck masses in pediatric patients have some preference for specific locations, with others being transpatial, a detailed knowledge of the head and neck spaces is necessary. Furthermore, given the importance of correctly naming these entities, it is crucial to be familiar with the most recent nomenclature.

To guide the readers toward differential diagnosis and correctly identify the mimics and pitfalls, we propose a pattern recognition approach focused on radiological findings, localization, and clinical characteristics. We will try to provide a step-by-step method for the radiological diagnosis

of the common head and neck masses, suggesting imaging protocols and key elements for the differential diagnosis.

IMAGING PROTOCOLS

The imaging modality of choice for head and neck masses in children is MR imaging. Computed tomography (CT) is, however, often needed in urgent settings/acute clinical presentation, in cases of aggressive masses such as rhabdomyosarcomas (RMSs) or lesions centered in the bone, to identify the extent of the bony destruction and guide the reconstructive surgery.[1,2] Furthermore, in some cases, the associated osseous changes help in the differential diagnosis such as cortical destruction with periosteal elevation and possible presence of gas in infection, expansion and thinning in benign processes, and aggressive destruction

[a] Department of Radiology, Neuroradiology Unit, Great Ormond Street Hospital, Great Ormond Street, London WC1N 3JH, UK; [b] Department of Advanced Biomedical Sciences, University of Naples "Federico II", Via Sergio Pansini 5, Naples 80131, Italy
* Corresponding author.
E-mail address: lorenzo.ugga@unina.it

Neuroimag Clin N Am 32 (2022) 433–445
https://doi.org/10.1016/j.nic.2022.02.003
1052-5149/22/© 2022 Elsevier Inc. All rights reserved.

> **Box 1**
> **Suggested MR protocol for head and neck masses assessment in children.**
>
> Key sequences:
>
> - Axial and coronal T2-weighted with fat saturation
> - Axial T1-weighted
> - Axial T2-weighted
> - Axial DWI
> - Postcontrast axial and coronal T1-weighted with fat saturation.
>
> Optional sequences:
>
> - MR angiography
> - MRV
> - Sagittal high-resolution T2-weighted
> - Coronal nonechoplanar DWI

in malignant processes.[3,4] Given the higher contrast resolution for soft tissues, we think that MR imaging should always be preferred to CT as a modality of choice in the evaluation of pediatric head and neck masses, and to avoid radiation risk in children.[5,6] Superficial masses may be initially studied with ultrasound providing useful information that are complementary to cross-section findings.[7,8]

Regarding the correct MR imaging protocol, a few basic differences between standard brain images and pediatric head and neck scans need to be clarified[9]:

1. Soft tissues of the head and neck have a large amount of fat, which can be used to the radiologist's advantage. A mass will show, in most of the cases, relative T2 hyperintense signal, relative T1 hypointense signal, and, at least in case of neoplasms and infections, contrast enhancement.
2. Thus, T2-weighted images (WIs) should be fat-saturated (eg,: short tau inversion recovery [STIR] or other similar techniques to suppress the fat signal) to distinguish the hyperintense neoplasm from normal tissue.
3. On the other hand, precontrast T1-WI should be acquired without fat saturation so the hyperintense fat is used as "passive contrast" surrounding the hypointense mass.
4. Finally, at least one postcontrast T1-WI should be acquired with fat saturation to separate the potential enhancing lesions from normal tissue.
5. Diffusion-weighted images (DWIs) can be useful to distinguish aggressive masses showing low apparent diffusion coefficient (ADC) values, indicative of high cellularity from benign processes *.
6. Pearl: it may be helpful to add a postcontrast T1-weighted sequence without fat saturation on the same plan as the precontrast T1-WI, to have the same sequence preinjection and post-injection of gadolinium and better define the anatomic characteristic of a lesion.
7. Additional MR imaging sequences for the study of head and neck masses in children, in specific cases, include:
   - magnetic resonance angiography to identify the presence of arteriovenous malformations (AVMs) and distinguish those from hemangiomas
   - coronal nonechoplanar DWI in case of suspected cholesteatoma of the temporal bone

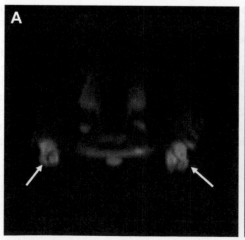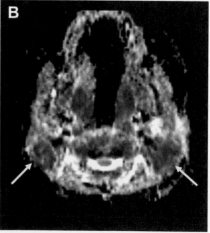

Fig. 1. MR imaging of normal neck nodes. Infant with normal lymph nodes showing high DWI signal (*A*) and relatively low ADC values (*B*) in the neck nodes bilaterally (*arrows*).

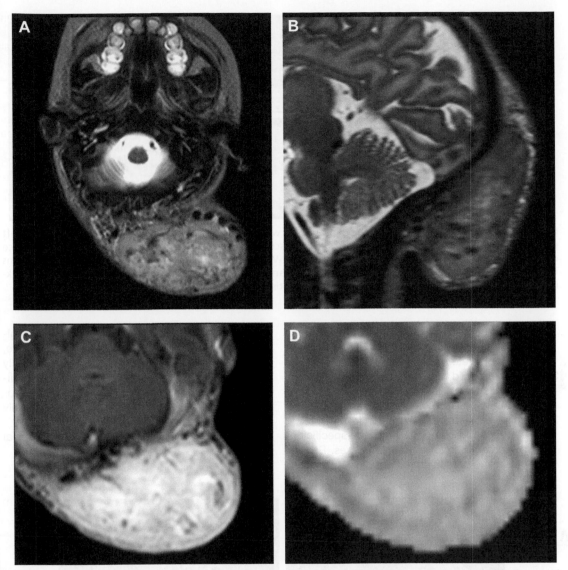

Fig. 2. Infantile hemangioma in the occipital subcutaneous soft tissue. Axial (*A*) and sagittal (*B*) T2-WI show multiple internal flow voids and intermediate T2-WI signal. Postcontrast axial T1-WI and axial ADC map (*C, D*) show homogeneous enhancement and high ADC values in keeping with low cellularity.

- MR venography (MRV) to exclude venous thrombosis
- sagittal high-resolution T2-WI in case of midline masses and to check for intracranial extension, typically in the case of nasal dermoid/epidermoid with sinus tracts.

A summary of the suggested MR protocol is shown in **Box 1**.

*An important pitfall in the use of DWI in the head and neck is related to some degree of physiologic DWI restriction of the lymph nodes because of their high cell density (**Fig. 1**), although some cut-offs have been proposed in literature mainly regarding the adult population to distinguish between metastatic and benign nodes.[10,11]

FIRST STEPS: A FEW BASIC QUESTIONS TO ASK YOURSELF WHEN APPROACHING A PEDIATRIC HEAD AND NECK MASS

To guide the reader in the differential diagnosis of main pediatric head and neck masses, we suggest starting from a few basic questions that can narrow down the range of possible entities.

1. Can I identify a discrete mass?

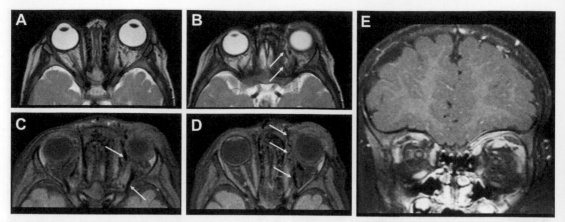

Fig. 3. Orbital AVM. Axial T2-WI (*A, B*) and axial T1-WI with fat saturation (*C, D*) in a 1-year-old male with left proptosis show multiple flow voids (*arrows*) without discrete mass identified, suggesting an AVM. The absence of enhancing solid tissue is confirmed on postcontrast T1-WI with fat saturation (*E*). Note the technical limitations in this scan with T2-WI acquired without fat saturation and precontrast T1-WI acquired with fat-saturation making it difficult to distinguish the presence of abnormal tissue in the background of orbital fat.

- Inflammatory processes and some vascular malformations such as AVM do not present with a discrete mass.
2. Is the mass solid, cystic, or mixed?
  - This allows an initial screening to narrow down the possible differential diagnoses.
3. In which neck space is the lesion located?
  - There is, to some extent, space-specificity for pediatric head and neck masses. RMSs and venous malformations tend to be

centered in the masticator space, hemangiomas in the subcutaneous soft tissue, lymphatic malformation (LM) are typically transpatial. However, in several cases, pediatric neck masses may occur in different locations than those they are classically associated with.
4. Does the lesion show aggressive radiological behavior?

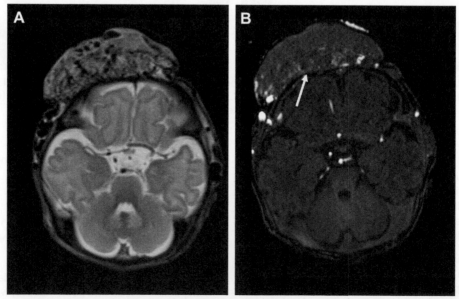

Fig. 4. Neonate with a rapidly involuting congenital hemangioma (RICH). Axial T2 (*A*) shows multiple serpiginous flow voids within a large mass, thus compatible with hemangioma rather than AVM, where a discrete mass is not expected. MRA (*B*) shows the absence of arterial flow signal in most of the vessels within the lesion (*arrow*) and no arteriovenous shunt in the sagittal sinus.

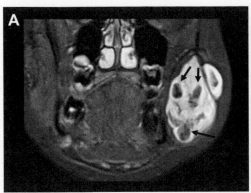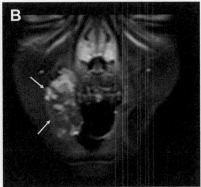

Fig. 5. Venous malformation in the left masseter. Coronal T2-WI with fat saturation (*A*) shows a markedly T2 hyperintense lesion with multiple internal areas of hypointensity in keeping with phleboliths (*black arrows*). Coronal T1-WI with fat saturation in another patient with confirmed venous malformation (*B*) shows the typical heterogeneous enhancement (*white arrows*), very different from the homogenous enhancement seen in hemangiomas.

- Bony erosion, nodal metastases, invasion of the surrounding soft tissues, and so forth, are associated with malignancies.
5. What are the characteristics of enhancement and DWI signal?
6. Is there any specific radiological hallmark?
7. What are the clinical characteristics associated with the mass?
   - Appearance of the overlying skin, progression or regression over time, signs of associated infection, and so forth, are important clues to the imaging differential.

The following sections focus on different radiological hallmarks useful for a pattern recognition approach to pediatric head and neck masses.

FLOW VOIDS AND MIMICS WITHIN THE LESION

The term "flow void" refers to signal loss particularly evident on T2-WI due to relatively fast movement of blood (or other fluids such as cerebrospinal fluid).[12] Multiple, serpiginous flow voids present in the head or neck spaces on MR imaging suggest the presence of multiple, anomalous blood vessels.

When serpiginous flow voids are noted in a pediatric head and neck mass, there are two main differential diagnoses that must be taken into account: hemangioma and AVM. Hemangiomas are benign vascular neoplasms divided into infantile type and congenital type, whereas AVMs are high-flow vascular malformations.[13]

Pearl: Multiple flow voids within a discrete and homogeneously enhancing mass suggest a hemangioma (**Fig. 2**); the presence of abnormal flow voids without a discrete mass is typical of AVM (**Fig. 3**).[14]

Other important elements in favor of hemangioma are:
1. typical reddish/pink flat appearance

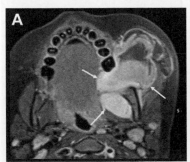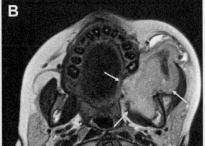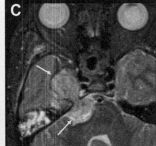

Fig. 6. Rhabdomyosarcoma of the masticator space. Axial postcontrast T1-WI with fat saturation and axial T2-WI (*A* and *B*, respectively) showing an RMS presenting as heterogeneous mass with bony erosion centered in the left masticator space (*arrows*). Axial T2-WI with fat saturation in another patient with parameningeal right masticator space RMS shows invasion of the right Meckel's cave, V3, and trigeminal cisternal segment (*C*).

Table 1
Summary of the radiological characteristics useful for the differential diagnosis between hemangioma, AVM, and venous malformations

Lesion	Flow Voids	Enhancement	Discrete Mass	T2-WI	Clinical Features
Hemangioma	YES	Homogeneous	YES	↑	Reddish, involution over time
AVM	YES	NO	NO	NO [b]	Worsening/bony lysis
Venous malformation	NO[a]	Heterogeneous	YES	↑↑	Bluish, slow growth over time

[a] Rounded T2 hypointense phleboliths may be present.
[b] Inflammation of the involved tissues is possible.

2. initial growth after birth followed by regression over time in the case of the more frequent infantile hemangioma
3. absent bony destruction
4. absence of nidus and arterialized veins expected in cases of arteriovenous shunt (**Fig. 4**)
5. T2-WI intermediate to hyperintense signal, homogeneous enhancement, absence of diffusion restriction, and well-defined borders (see **Fig. 2**).

Pitfall (I): Congenital hemangiomas are present at birth, whereas infantile hemangiomas develop after birth and include rapidly involuting congenital hemangiomas, noninvoluting congenital hemangiomas, and partially involuting congenital hemangiomas. They have similar dermatologic appearances to congenital hemangioma but have a different trajectory over time.[15]

Pitfall (II): Presence of T2 hypointense calcifications (phleboliths, typical of venous malformations) or internal fibrotic bundles can be mistaken for flow voids. However, phleboliths have a typical round appearance without a serpiginous shape. Furthermore, venous malformations are very bright on T2-WI, higher signal than hemangiomas, demonstrate heterogeneous enhancement, and often are located in the masticator space[14] (**Fig. 5**).

Table 1 summarizes the radiological findings useful for the differential diagnosis between hemangioma, AVM, and venous malformations.

OTHER COMMON SOLID HEAD AND NECK MASSES IN CHILDREN

If there is a solid mass without flow voids or phleboliths, the differential diagnosis is based on location, presence of aggressive behavior toward the surrounding soft tissues/bones, and clinical characteristics (age, sex, symptoms, evolution over time).

The most common aggressive tumors in the head and neck region in children are RMSs. Main pearls for the differential diagnosis are:

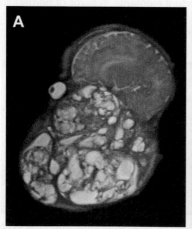
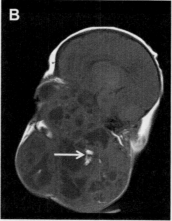
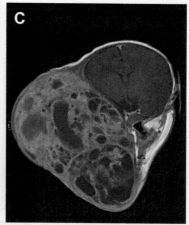

Fig. 7. Neonatal teratoma. Sagittal T2-WI (*A*), T1-WI and coronal postcontrast T1-WI (*C*) in a neonate showing large heterogeneous, solid-cystic teratoma with fatty areas demonstrated on precontrast T1-WI (*arrow in B*) and marked enhancement of the solid portion. There is distortion of the surrounding structures with compromise of the airways.

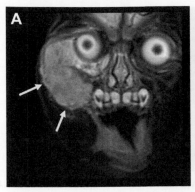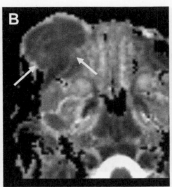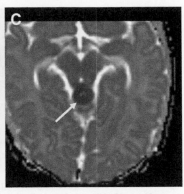

Fig. 8. Periorbital malignant rhabdoid tumor in an infant with SMARCB1 mutation. Coronal T2-WI with fat saturation shows invasion of the surrounding soft tissue (*arrows* in *A*), whereas axial ADC map demonstrates low values due to high cellularity (*arrows* in *B*). Another mass in the same patient showing diffusion restriction is seen in the supravermian cistern (*arrow* in *C*) is in keeping with an embryonal tumor also caused by SMARCB1 mutation.

- the age of the patient: RMSs present between 2 and 5 years old or in young adults (15 to 19 years old)
- the localization: RMSs show predilection for the masticator space
- aggressive radiological behavior.

Pearl (I): Typical radiological appearance of an RMS in the region of head and neck include a heterogeneously enhancing mass, with internal areas of necrosis, centered in the masticator space and with erosion of the contiguous bones. Furthermore, imaging features favoring an RMS are diffusion restriction and avid fluorodeoxyglucose (FDG)-positron emission tomography (PET) uptake[4,16] (**Fig. 6**).

Pearl (II): Parameningeal RMSs can involve the cranial nerves with different mechanisms compared to the adult head and neck carcinomas.[4] The use of high-resolution sequences to better visualize the cranial nerve involvement should be considered in these cases.

USEFULNESS OF AGE IN THE DIFFERENTIAL DIAGNOSIS

RMSs are rare in infants and neonates; thus, other entities need to be considered in the case of solid masses in younger children. These are:

- Teratoma: Solid-cystic mass in neonates (also often congenital and visible on fetal scans) characterized by heterogeneous enhancement, cystic components, and internal fatty areas (**Fig. 7**).
- Malignant rhabdoid tumors of the head and neck region: Very aggressive radiological features including diffusion restriction, necrosis, and bony erosion, and characterized by SMARCB1 mutation[17,18] (**Fig. 8**).
- Hairy polyp: Also known as fibrovascular polyp. Benign tumors in infants and neonates, involving the naso-oropharynx and characterized radiologically by a fibrovascular central stalk surrounded by fat (**Fig. 9**).[19,20]

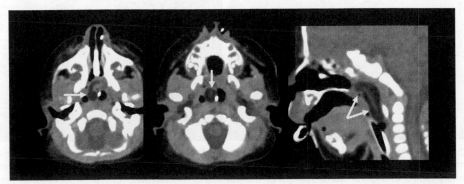

Fig. 9. Hairy polyp on CT. There is a polypoid mass arising from the nasopharynx in this neonate; characterized by a dense fibrovascular stalk surrounded by fat (*arrows*).

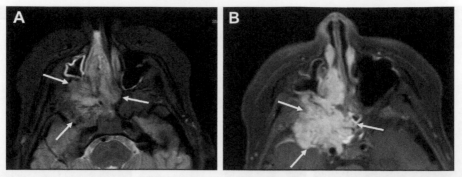

Fig. 10. Juvenile nasopharyngeal angiofibroma. A teenaged male with typical location and appearance of a JNA (*arrows*) on T2-WI with fat saturation (*A*) and postcontrast T1-WI (*B*) demonstrating avid enhancement and prominent internal flow voids.

- Sialoblastoma: Aggressive mass presenting in neonates, often located in the parotid space.[21]

Pearl (III): Patients with SMARCB1 mutation can develop synchronous intracranial neoplasms such as atypical teratoid rhabdoid tumor, pinealoblastoma, and malignant rhabdoid tumors (see **Fig. 9**C).

Juvenile nasopharyngeal angiofibroma (JNA) is almost exclusively seen in adolescent males and has a very typical appearance of a lobulated, hypervascular enhancing mass, centered in the sphenopalatine foramen, extending in the nasal cavity and in the pterygopalatine fossa (**Fig. 10**). The mass is locally aggressive; CT and

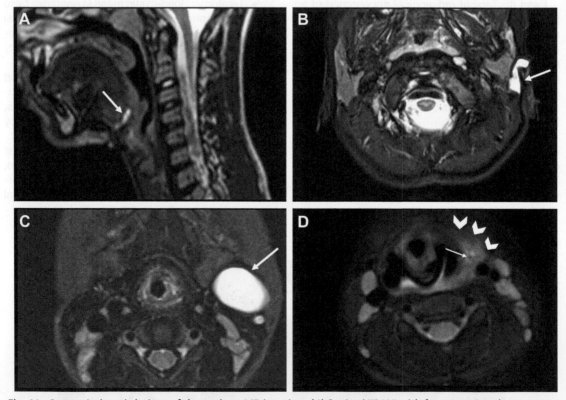

Fig. 11. Congenital cystic lesions of the neck on MR imaging. (*A*) Sagittal T2-WI with fat saturation shows a recurrence of thyroglossal duct cyst in the floor of mouth with discharge from midline sinus (*arrow*); (*B*) first branchial cleft anomaly type 2 along the lateral margin of the parotid gland (*arrow*); (*C*) typical location of second branchial cleft anomaly in the neck (*arrow*); and (*D*) inflammatory tissue adjacent to the thyroid gland on the left (*arrowheads*) with small tract within it (*arrow*) in keeping with fourth branchial cleft anomaly.

angiography are necessary to demonstrate bony involvement (mainly expansion) and vascularization for preoperative planning.

Pitfall: JNAs also contain internal flow voids because of the high vascularity; however, the typical age, sex, and location pose no problem in differentiating from hemangioma or AVM.

DIFFERENTIAL DIAGNOSIS OF PEDIATRIC CYSTIC HEAD AND NECK MASSES

Cystic lesions in the head and neck region all have similar radiological characteristics: a thin cystic wall (often enhancing and smooth) and internal core that follows the water signal on all sequences and water attenuation on CT.

The differential diagnosis of simple cysts is based mainly on location, with an underlying embryologic basis (Table 2).[8,22–25]

Pearl (I): A cyst may be infected and being associated with inflammation of the surrounding soft tissues, thickening of the cyst wall, and inflammatory symptoms.

Pitfall: The embryologic origin of the so-called third and fourth branchial cleft anomalies is still debated, and the radiological findings may overlap. It has been speculated that left-sided inflammatory neck tissue involving the thyroid gland and with a sinus opening in the pyriform fossa (infected fourth or third branchial cleft anomalies) may actually originate from the embryonal thymopharyngeal duct of the third branchial pouch.[26]

Cystic pediatric head and neck masses with different imaging characteristics

- Pyogenic abscesses are characterized by a core of pus showing marked diffusion restriction and symptoms related to the infection[27]
- Dermoid/epidermoid are cysts that can show variable signal intensity on T1-WIs depending on the fat content of the lesion and diffusion restriction in case of keratin-filled cyst. As both can have the same radiological characteristics, including DWI high signal,[28] and the histologic differentiation may also be challenging, we suggest that those entities should be reported as *dermoid/epidermoid* rather than trying to distinguish between the two.
- LMs (Fig. 12): radiological key features are T2 hyperintensity, fluid-fluid levels, and no-enhancement (apart from the thin enhancing wall). These masses are typically transpatial (involving several neck spaces). These are part of the vascular malformations and should no longer be called cystic hygromas.[14,29] Furthermore, LMs can be microcystic or macrocystic,[30] depending on the size of the fluid-

Table 2
Location-based differential diagnosis of pediatric simple cysts in the head and neck region

Entity	Location
Thyroglossal duct cyst (Fig. 12A)	• Midline/paramedian between foramen caecum at tongue base and thyroid gland • Typically embedded in the strap muscles
Vallecular cyst	• Within the vallecula • Pushes the epiglottis against the wall of the pharynx
Foregut duplication cyst	• In the anterior third of the tongue as opposed to thyroglossal duct cyst and vallecular cyst • Can be serpiginous
First branchial cleft anomaly (Fig. 12B)	• Posteroinferior to the auricle (type 1) • Adjacent to parotid gland (type 2)
Second branchial cleft anomaly (Fig. 12C)	• Anteromedial to the SCM muscle (superior 1/3) • Posterior to submandibular gland • Lateral to the carotid space
Third branchial cleft anomaly	• Posterior to the SCM muscle (inferior 2/3) • In the posterior cervical space
Fourth branchial cleft cyst (Fig. 12D)	• Often tract between the pyriform sinus and the thyroid gland • Left +++ • Often infected

Abbreviation: SCM, sternocleidomastoid.

filled part of the lesion. In macrocystic LMs, cysts measure more than 2 cm in diameter, whereas microcystic LMs are made up of smaller cysts or do not present a cystic component and for this reason may simulate a solid enhancing neoplasm.

Pitfall (II): Aneurysmal bone cysts (ABC) are also characterized by typical fluid-fluid levels

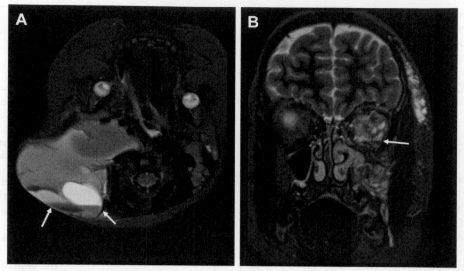

Fig. 12. Lymphatic malformation on MR imaging. Macrocystic (A) and microcystic (B) lymphatic malformations are seen on T2-WI with fat saturation. Note the presence of fluid-fluid levels due to internal bleeding in both (arrows) and the involvement of several spaces of the head and neck. In particular, the microcystic lymphatic malformation shows orbital, masticator, and scalp components.

and can be seen in the head and neck region but are typically located in the bone, which allows the differential diagnosis with LM (Fig. 13).[31]

PITFALLS RELATED TO BONY MASSES IN THE SKULL AND SKULL BASE

Apart from ABC, other lesions typically centered in the skull or skull base in children are:

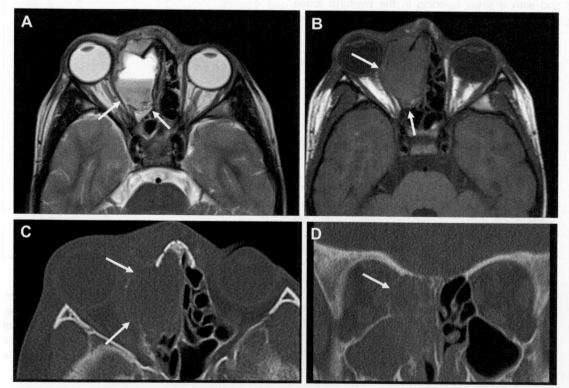

Fig. 13. Aneurysmal bone cyst. Expansile cystic lesion with fluid-fluid levels centered in the ethmoid bone (arrows) on axial T2-WI (A), axial T1-WI (B), and CT (axial: C and coronal: D).

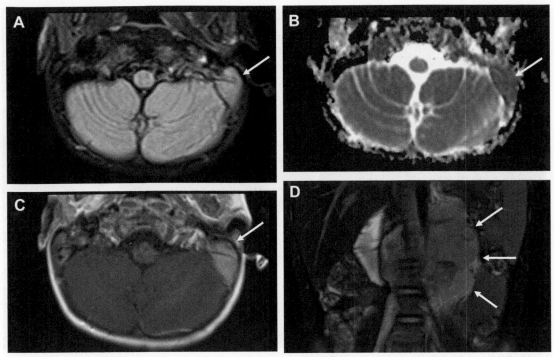

Fig. 14. Neuroblastoma metastasis. Axial FLAIR (*A*), axial ADC map (*B*), and postcontrast T1-WI (*C*) showing isolated, enhancing, and diffusion restricting mass in the left temporal bone (*arrows*) of a 29-month-old male. The mass was originally diagnosed as possible LCH, but the diffusion restriction and the young age of the patient prompted an abdominal ultrasound and MR imaging that confirmed a neuroblastoma (*arrows* in *D*) and avoided unnecessary biopsy.

1. Neuroblastoma metastases: bony lesions are much more common than nodal or intracranial metastases
2. Langerhans cells histiocytosis (LCH).

In a very young child with DWI restricting mass lesions in the skull or skull base, the next step is an abdominal ultrasound to exclude a primary neuroblastoma. This is particularly important to avoid unnecessary biopsy and to hasten appropriate management (**Fig. 14**).

If there are single or multiple lytic skull lesions without sclerotic rim and beveled edge, associated radiological findings of LCH need to be investigated, namely vertebra plana (flattened vertebral bodies), white matter lesions in the brain, pituitary or infundibular mass, or absent posterior pituitary T1-WI "bright spot" (**Fig. 15**).[32,33]

Pearl (I): Both LCH and metastatic neuroblastoma can involve the temporal bone.

Pearl (II): Neuroblastomas typically show a permeative destruction of the bone on CT and

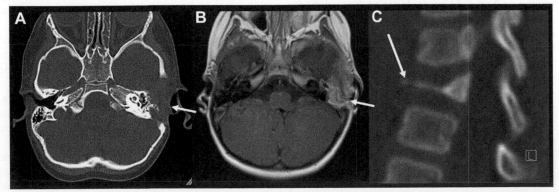

Fig. 15. Langerhans cell histiocytosis. Axial CT (*A*), axial postcontrast T1-WI showing an enhancing destructive LCH lesion in the temporal bone (*arrows* in *A* and *B*). Sagittal CT reformat shows vertebra plana (*arrow* in *C*).

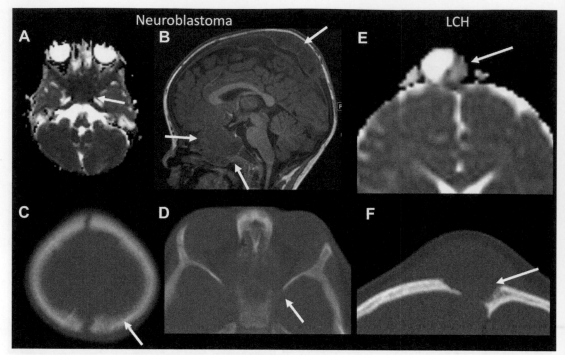

Fig. 16. DWI and CT differences between LCH and neuroblastoma. ADC map (*A*) and sagittal T1-WI (*B*) in a patient with metastatic neuroblastoma show striking diffusion restriction and large masses in the vaults and skull base (*arrows*). CT scan in the same patient (*C* and *D*) demonstrates permeative destruction of the bone. ADC map (*E*) and CT (*F*) in a patient with confirmed LCH show intermediate or high ADC values and a lytic lesion. One should be aware that a radiological overlap between these entities is possible.

striking diffusion restriction. LCH presents with sharp lytic lesions and intermediate ADC value, although on DWI they can simulate high cellularity in some cases (**Fig. 16**).[34]

Pearl (III): In lesions in the skull, CT provides complementary information to MR imaging and MR protocol with fat-saturated T2-WI and post-contrast T1-WI should be acquired.[35]

SUMMARY

A complete knowledge of the radiological hallmarks of specific entities such as flow voids, phleboliths or fluid-fluid levels, location (especially for cystic masses), and epidemiologic characteristics can help the radiologist in the differential diagnosis between different pediatric head and neck lesions. We stressed several pearls and pitfalls that can guide the rigorous approach to these entities.

CLINICS CARE POINTS

- Basic knowledge of radiological appearances in pediatric head and neck masses.
- Focus on clinico-radiological correlations and elements of differential diagnosis.

- Extensive iconography with common and uncommon radiological characteristics of each entity.

DISCLOSURE

The authors have nothing to disclose.

REFERENCES

1. Freling Nicole JM, Merks JHM, Saeed P, et al. Imaging findings in craniofacial childhood rhabdomyosarcoma. Pediatr Radiol 2010;40(11):1723–38.
2. Eckardt AM, Barth EL, Berten J, et al. Pediatric mandibular resection and reconstruction: long-term results with autogenous rib grafts. Craniomaxillofac Trauma Reconstr 2010;3(1):25–32.
3. Zhu J, Zhang J, Tang G, et al. Computed tomography and magnetic resonance imaging observations of rhabdomyosarcoma in the head and neck. Oncol Lett 2014;8(1):155–60.
4. Talenti G, Picariello S, Robson C, et al. Magnetic resonance features and cranial nerve involvement in pediatric head and neck rhabdomyosarcomas. Neuroradiology 2021. https://doi.org/10.1007/s00234-021-02765-0.

5. Huda W, Vance A. Patient radiation doses from adult and pediatric {CT. Am J Roentgenol 2007;188(2):540–6.

6. Carrie P. Pediatric computed tomography scans: Weighing the risks and benefits: a new study suggests that computed tomography-related radiation may increase the risk of brain tumors, but the conversation, physicians say, is complex-and far from settled. Cancer 2019;125(2):171–3.

7. Junn Jacqueline C, Soderlund Karl A, Glastonbury Christine M. Imaging of head and neck cancer with {CT}, {MRI}, and {US. Semin Nucl Med 2021; 51(1):3–12.

8. Gupta Bansal Anmol, Rebecca Oudsema, Masseaux Joy A, et al. {US} of pediatric superficial masses of the head and neck. Radiographics 2018;38(4):1239–63.

9. Saunders Dawn E, Thompson C, Roxanne G, et al. Magnetic resonance imaging protocols for paediatric neuroradiology. Pediatr Radiol 2007;37(8): 789–97.

10. Anna P, Pietro G, Luciano I, et al. Diffusion-weighted {MRI} in cervical lymph nodes: differentiation between benign and malignant lesions. Eur J Radiol 2011;77(2):281–6.

11. Chen C, Lin Z, Xiao Y, et al. Role of diffusion-weighted imaging in the discrimination of benign and metastatic parotid area lymph nodes in patients with nasopharyngeal carcinoma. Sci Rep 2018;8(1):281.

12. Vlaardingerbroek Marinus T, den Boer Jacques A. Motion and flow. Magn. Reson. Imaging. Berlin (Heidelberg): Springer Berlin Heidelberg; 2003. p. 321–422.

13. Michel W, Francine B, Adams D, et al. Vascular anomalies classification: recommendations from the international society for the study of vascular anomalies. Pediatrics 2015;136(1):e203–14.

14. Steinklein JM, Shatzkes DR. Imaging of vascular lesions of the head and neck. Otolaryngol Clin North Am 2018;51(1):55–76.

15. North Paula E. Classification and pathology of congenital and perinatal vascular anomalies of the head and neck. Otolaryngol Clin North Am 2018; 51(1):1–39.

16. Norman G, Fayter D, Lewis-Light K, et al. An emerging evidence base for PET-CT in the management of childhood rhabdomyosarcoma: systematic review. BMJ Open 2015;5(1):e006030.

17. Wolfe Adam D, Capitini Christian M, Salamat Shahriar M, et al. Neck rhabdoid tumors: clinical features and consideration of autologous stem cell transplant. J Pediatr Hematol Oncol 2018;40(1):e50–4.

18. Abdullah A, Patel Y, Lewis TJ, et al. Extrarenal malignant rhabdoid tumors: radiologic findings with histopathologic correlation. Cancer Imaging 2010;10:97–101.

19. Tariq MU, Din NU, Bashir MR. Hairy polyp, a clinicopathologic study of four cases. Head Neck Pathol 2013;7(3):232–5.

20. Wu J, Schulte J, Yang C, et al. Hairy polyp of the nasopharynx arising from the eustachian tube. Head Neck Pathol 2016;10(2):213–6.

21. Choudhary K, Panda S, Beena VT, et al. Sialoblastoma: a literature review from 1966-2011. Natl J Maxillofac Surg 2013;4(1):13–8.

22. Kieran SM, Robson CD, Nosé V, et al. Foregut duplication cysts in the head and neck: presentation, diagnosis, and management. Arch Otolaryngol Neck Surg 2010;136(8):778–82.

23. Fastenberg J, Nassar M. First branchial cleft cyst. N Engl J Med 2016;375(16):e33.

24. LaPlante Justin K, Pierson Nicholas S, Hedlund Gary L. Common pediatric head and neck congenital/developmental anomalies. Radiol Clin North Am 2015;53(1):181–96.

25. Turkington JRA, Paterson A, Sweeney LE, et al. Neck masses in children. Br J Radiol 2005; 78(925):75–85.

26. Thomas B, Shroff M, Forte V, et al. Revisiting imaging features and the embryologic basis of third and fourth branchial anomalies. Am J Neuroradiol 2010;31(4):755–60.

27. Muccio CF, Caranci F, D'Arco F, et al. Magnetic resonance features of pyogenic brain abscesses and differential diagnosis using morphological and functional imaging studies: a pictorial essay. J Neuroradiol 2014;41(3):153–67.

28. Balasundaram P, Garg A, Prabhakar A, et al. Evolution of epidermoid cyst into dermoid cyst: Embryological explanation and radiological-pathological correlation. Neuroradiol J 2019;32(2):92–7.

29. White CL, Olivieri B, Restrepo R, et al. Low-flow vascular malformation pitfalls: from clinical examination to practical imaging evaluation–Part 1, lymphatic malformation mimickers. Am J Roentgenol 2016;206(5):940–51.

30. D'Arco F, Ugga L. Computed tomography and magnetic resonance imaging in pediatric salivary gland diseases: a guide to the differential diagnosis. Pediatr Radiol 2020;50(9):1293–307.

31. Fennessy BG, Vargas SO, Silvera MV, et al. Paediatric aneurysmal bone cysts of the head and neck. J Laryngol Otol 2009;123(6):635–41.

32. Stull MA, Kransdorf MJ, Devaney KO. Langerhans cell histiocytosis of bone. Radiographics 1992; 12(4):801–23.

33. Nicollas R, Rome A, Belaïch H, et al. Head and neck manifestation and prognosis of Langerhans' cell histiocytosis in children. Int J Pediatr Otorhinolaryngol 2010;74(6):669–73.

34. Ginat D, Mangla R, Yeaney G, et al. Diffusion-weighted imaging of skull lesions. J Neurol Surg B Skull Base 2014;75(03):204–13.

35. Ugga L, Cuocolo R, Cocozza S, et al. Spectrum of lytic lesions of the skull: a pictorial essay. Insights Imaging 2018;9(5):845–56.